T0220094

THE FEELING BRAIN

The Feeling Brain is one of a series of low-cost books
under the title PSYCHOANALYTIC IDEAS which brings together the best of
public lectures and other writings given by analysts of the British
Psycho-Analytical Society on important psychoanalytic subjects.

Series Editor: James Rose

THE FEELING BRAIN

Selected Papers on Neuropsychoanalysis

Mark Solms

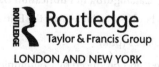

Routledge
Taylor & Francis Group

LONDON AND NEW YORK

First published 2015 by
Karnac Books Ltd.

Published 2018 by Routledge
2 Park Square, Milton Park, Abingdon, Oxon OX14 4RN
711 Third Avenue, New York, NY 10017, USA

Routledge is an imprint of the Taylor & Francis Group, an informa business

British Library Cataloguing in Publication Data

A C.I.P. for this book is available from the British Library

ISBN: 9781782202721 (pbk)

Edited, designed, and produced by Communication Crafts

CONTENTS

PART V
NEUROPSYCHOANALYTIC PERSPECTIVES
ON CONSCIOUSNESS

ABOUT THE AUTHOR AND CONTRIBUTORS

Mark Solms is the Chair of Neuropsychology at the University of Cape Town and Groote Schuur Hospital (Departments of Psychology and Neurology), President of the South African Psychoanalytical Association, and Research Chair of the International Psychoanalytical Association. He was awarded Honorary Membership of the New York Psychoanalytic Society in 1998 and the American College of Psychoanalysts in 2004 and will be named Honorary Fellow of the American College of Psychiatrists in 2016. He is best known for his discovery of the forebrain mechanisms of dreaming, and for his integration of psychoanalytic theories and methods with those of modern neuroscience. He founded the International Neuropsychoanalysis Society in 2000 and was Founding Editor of the journal *Neuropsychoanalysis*. He has published widely in both neuroscientific and psychoanalytic journals, as well as in general-interest publications such as *Scientific American*. He has published more than 250 articles and book chapters and 5 books. His second book, *The Neuropsychology of Dreams* (1997), was a landmark contribution to the field. Together with Oliver Turnbull he wrote *The Brain and the Inner World* (2002), which is a best-seller and has been translated into 12 languages. He is the authorized editor and translator of the forthcoming *Revised Standard Edition of the Complete Psychological Works of Sigmund Freud* (24 vols.) and the *Complete Neuroscientific Works of Sigmund Freud* (4 vols.).

Jaak Panksepp holds the Baily Endowed Chair of Animal Well-Being Science in the Neuroscience Program of Washington State University's College of Veterinary Medicine (Department of Integrative Physiology and Neuroscience) and is Emeritus Distinguished Research Professor of the Department of Psychology at Bowling Green State University. He is an internationally recognized pioneer in the neuro-affective study of emotions in mammals. He coined the term "affective neuroscience", the name for the field that studies the neural mechanisms of emotional behaviors and feelings, and he generated the first neural (opioid-addictive) model of social bonding as well as the first brain research on mammalian playfulness, with implications for the treatment of depression and ADHD, respectively. He is known for his research on laughter in non-human animals, which has yielded another antidepressant currently in human testing. He is author of *Affective Neuroscience: The Foundations of Human and Animal Emotions* (1998) and *The Archaeology of Mind: The Neuroevolutionary Origins of Human Emotions"* (2012). He is especially fond of the "White Star Award for National Service" from the Estonian Government.

Eleni Pantelis is the Senior Clinical Coordinator of the Masters Neuropsychology Programme at the University of Cape Town. She is currently completing her PhD, researching human homologues of basic-emotion command systems identified in other mammals.

Oliver H. Turnbull is a neuropsychologist and clinical psychologist. He is a Professor of Neuropsychology and Pro Vice-Chancellor in Bangor University, UK. He was for many years the Editor of the journal *Neuropsychoanalysis* and Secretary of the International Neuropsychoanalysis Society. His interests include emotion-based learning, and the experience that we describe as "intuition"; the role of emotion in false beliefs, especially in neurological patients; and the neuroscience of psychotherapy. He is the author of a number of scientific articles on these topics, and (together with Mark Solms) of the popular science text *The Brain and the Inner World* (2002).

FOREWORD

This book is a compilation of a number of papers on the matter of neuropsychoanalysis. Being a major contributor in the development of this new branch of psychoanalysis, Mark Solms is well placed to offer an authoritative introduction to those unfamiliar with it. A summary of what he will discuss is made in his Introduction, and it includes a consideration of the origins of this enquiry and research into its implications for the understanding of some neurological and psychiatric disorders. He continues by considering dreams and the fundamental problem of consciousness. His description of the development and application of these new concepts makes a valuable contribution to the fundamental question of how we can be objective about subjectivity.

James Rose
Series Editor
Psychoanalytic Ideas

Introduction

The term "neuropsychoanalysis" means different things to different people. To some, like Blass and Carmeli (2007), it is a dangerous term—referring to something un-psychoanalytic, if not anti-analytic—an approach to the mind that misses the point of (and thereby undermines) what psychoanalysis is all about. Psychoanalysis is about meaning-making, personal meaning-making, and is therefore an intrinsically hermeneutic and subjective discipline. It can never be a natural science, as neuroscience is. To these commentators, adding the epithet "neuro-" to "psychoanalysis" is therefore an oxymoron. What it really means is psychoanalysis minus the psyche, psychoanalysis biologized and reduced to neuroscience, with psychoanalysis being eliminated in the process. To others, neuropsychoanalysis promises (or threatens—see Ramus, 2013) to be the salvation of psychoanalysis. It is an approach to the dynamics of the mind that has the potential to rid the discipline of its ideological baggage, of its reputation for being a closed system of beliefs rather than an evidence-based body of knowledge. To these commentators, the personality is just a part of nature, and there should be no reason why it, like the rest of nature, cannot be reduced to natural scientific laws. Moreover, the laws governing the development and functions of the human personality must surely, somehow be reconcilable with the laws governing these aspects of the human brain; since who can deny that the brain is the organ of the mind—that these two things (mind and brain) are ultimately the same part of nature?

Part I of this book—a book that aims to introduce neuropsychoanalysis to a general readership—addresses this polemic by way of three chapters that try to explain, in different ways, what I mean by the term. My starting point is that psychoanalysis, in its essence, has *always* straddled the divide between these two apparently antithetical approaches. Freud, who was a neuroscientist and clinical neurologist, wrote in his and Breuer's *Studies on Hysteria* (Freud, 1895d) that:

> It still strikes me myself as strange that the case histories I write should read like short stories and that, as one might say, they lack the serious stamp of science. I must console myself with the reflection that the nature of the subject is evidently responsible for this, rather than any preference of my own. [p. 160]

He went on:

> The fact is that . . . a detailed description of mental processes such as we are accustomed to find in the works of imaginative writers enables me, with the use of a few psychological formulas, to obtain at least some kind of insight into the course of that affliction. [p. 161]

What Freud meant by "insight into the course of the illness" was knowledge of the causal chain of events by which the affliction comes about. But the operative phrase is: "with the use of a few psychological formulas". For what if the formulas are wrong? Freud was the first to admit this possibility. That is why he revised the formulas he used in his *Studies* with Breuer and replaced them with others—in fact, with a series of others—from 1895 right up to the last papers he wrote at the time of his death in 1939.

This much seems obvious. Psychoanalytic formulas (explanatory assumptions) have always been open to revision on the basis of new evidence. But the critics of neuropsychoanalysis go further. They object to the *kind* of evidence that we neuropsychoanalysts use when considering theoretical and technical revisions. Here they rest their case on Freud's assertion that "the nature of the subject is evidently responsible for . . . [our reliance on descriptions] such as we are accustomed to find in the works of imaginative writers". In short, according to these commentators, to make inferences about the human subject on the basis of objective, physical data is to overlook the proper evidential base of psychoanalysis. An absolutely essential property of the mind, as opposed to its bodily organ, is that it is "first and last . . . a subject, not an object" (Sacks, 1998, p. 177). I readily concede this point. In fact, I myself have often quoted Sacks's felicitous phrase. The very starting point of neuropsychoanalysis (in the mid-1980s) was my conviction *as a neuropsychologist* that the science of our time does not take sufficient account of "the nature of the subject".

However, we also have to take account of Freud's remark to the effect that:

> Biology is a land of unlimited possibilities. We cannot guess what answers it will return in a few dozen years. They may be of a kind that will blow away the whole artificial structure of our hypotheses. [1920g, p. 60]

What Freud referred to here is the fact that the mind may be first and last a subject, but it is also undeniably embodied. Freud's great contribution sprang from his recognition that mental life is unavoidably tethered to the body, and thereby to biology. There can be no mind without body. This is why Freud is described as a "Biologist of the Mind" (Sulloway, 1979). In fact, according to Freud, the very existence of the mind—of a sentient instrument for learning how to meet our vital and reproductive needs in the world—is a product of evolutionary biological forces (Freud, 1911b). The mind is not exempt from the laws of natural selection. Hence the great importance of sexuality in the life of the mind.

In short, what is unique about the part of nature we are concerned with in psychoanalysis is that it is *both* an object *and* a subject. *This simple fact is the starting point of all neuropsychoanalysis.* On this basis, neuropsychoanalysis seeks to *link* the findings of the science of the mind as an object with those of the mind as a subject. It is an approach to the mind that recognizes this unique, dualistic realization. But it makes absolutely no attempt to reduce the one realization to the other. Rather, it is a serious, systematic attempt to reconcile the two aspects of the mind with each other. I do not see how else we can proceed.

My justification for this approach, and some of its implications, then, form the stuff of the first three chapters in this book. Readers seeking more neuropsychologically or neuroscientifically oriented approaches to the issues covered in these publications, which were written for psychoanalytic, psychological, and engineering audiences, respectively, may fruitfully consult Turnbull and Solms (2007) or Panksepp and Solms (2012).

Part II illustrates what happens when one takes this point of view seriously *within neurology*. I trust the publications that make up this section will put paid to any lingering doubts about my trying to reduce psychoanalysis to neuroscience. I selected these publications in order to show what I mean when I say that the very starting point of neuropsychoanalysis was my conviction that the neuroscience of our time does not take sufficient account of the nature of the subject.

The first chapter in this section, "Is the Brain More Real Than the Mind?" (chapter 4), puts clinical meat on the bones of some of the philosophical arguments set out in Part I. It also begins to illustrate the benefits for behavioural neurology and neuropsychology of doing so. While this is not the main focus of this chapter, it also describes some findings about the functions of the right cerebral hemisphere that emerge from a psychoanalytic study of patients with damage to this part of the brain. That is, it demonstrates what happens when one takes seriously the notion that the right hemisphere is, as it were, not only an object but also a subject. Readers seeking a more thoroughgoing and direct treatment of these findings, with particular emphasis on the syndrome of anosognosia, should consult Solms (1999) (also reported in Kaplan-Solms & Solms, 2000; see also Turnbull, Fotopoulou, & Solms, in press).

The next chapter (chapter 5) also focuses on the psychoanalytic study of a mental disorder arising from damage to a particular brain region—in this instance, the disorder known as confabulatory amnesia. I think this chapter, essentially a case study, illustrates particularly well what I mean when I say that neuropsychoanalysis tries to build bridges between the two approaches to the mind—

namely, subjective meaning-making and objective anatomy. I hope it demonstrates how these two approaches can be seamlessly reconciled, using the clinico-anatomical method—a method that I have always considered to be the preeminent neuropsychoanalytic method. As in chapter 4, I attempt here to show what new light is cast on a neurological disorder when it is considered from the psychoanalytic point of view; but I also try in this chapter to show how the neuropsychoanalytic approach makes it possible to begin to locate within the tissues of the brain some of the metapsychological abstractions that Freud derived from his work with purely psychiatric disorders. In doing so, this aspect of the chapter puts further meat on the bones of some of the epistemological and methodological arguments set out in Part I. More technical reports, which will be of interest only to neuroscientifically educated readers, are: Feinberg, De Luca, Giacino, Roane, & Solms, (2005), Fotopoulou, Conway, and Solms (2007), Fotopoulou, Conway, Solms, Tyrer, and Kopelman (2008), Fotopoulou, Conway, Tyrer, et al. (2008), and Fotopoulou, Solms, and Turnbull (2004).

I have said that I consider the clinico-anatomical method to be the preeminent neuropsychoanalytic method, but it is by no means the only method that may legitimately be described as neuropsychoanalytic. In Part III, made up of two accessible publications that exemplify neuropsychoanalytic perspectives on some psychiatric (as opposed to neurological) disorders, I try to show how this approach can cast new light on old hypotheses, using different methods of investigation. Here I am referring mainly to combined psychoanalytic and psychopharmacological methods, although these two chapters do not report directly on studies in which we made psychoanalytic observations on cases where specific neurotransmitters were manipulated (for an example of this type of research, see Pantelis & Solms, 2007). The principle upon which such studies are based is exactly the same as for the clinico-anatomical method, except that in this case the "anatomical" side of the equation (studying psychoanalytically the effects of a brain lesion) is replaced with a "physiological" side (studying psychoanalytically the effects of a neuropharmacological intervention).

The two publications making up this section, focusing on depression (chapter 6) and addiction (chapter 7), rather than demonstrating the clinico-physiological (or clinico-pharmaco-logical) method, illustrate the relationship between neuropsy-choanalysis and psychopharmacology more generally. The neuropsychoanalytic approach to psychopharmacology is quite different from the psychiatric approach. It is not sufficiently widely appreciated how little psychopharmacological research is theory-driven—that is, how little it derives from any understand-ing of the psychological functions of the neurotransmitter and neuromodulator systems of the human brain. Almost all (liter-ally, all) drugs currently used in psychiatry were discovered by accident; post-hoc explanations were then given for their effects. That is how we arrived at such absurd notions as the claim that depression results from serotonin deficiency. The thinking goes like this: if serotonin reuptake inhibitors (which increase sero-tonin levels in the brain) happen to reduce depression, then depression must be caused by too little serotonin. Simple as that! The neuropsychoanalytic approach, by contrast, is rooted in a theory-driven approach to the emotional brain known as "affec-tive neuroscience" (Panksepp, 1998a). Affective neuroscience is based mainly in animal research, in which the emotional effects of various experimental manipulations (ablations, electrical stim-ulations, etc.) are systematically observed in order to discern the basic affective circuitry of the mammalian brain. Since such cir-cuits are so fundamental (with emotion being such a basic brain function), they are conserved in human beings. The role of neu-ropsychoanalysis, then, is to extrapolate from the animal models to human beings, in whom electrical stimulation experiments and so forth cannot be so easily performed. Since, on the other hand, humans have the unique ability to report verbally on their sub-jective states, this extrapolation works both ways, and the human studies act as an important restraint on inferences derived from animal observation. (To their credit, affective neuroscientists start from the assumption that other animals, like us, *do have* affective experiences; see Panksepp & Solms, 2012.) The massive implica-tions of this line of research for psychoanalysis, and especially for psychoanalytic affect and drive theory, have only just begun to be explored (see Panksepp, 1999; Panksepp & Biven, 2012; Solms & Nersessian 1999; Wright & Panksepp, 2012).

I hope that chapters 6 and 7 serve to illustrate the deep and ever-growing relationship that exists between neuropsychoanalysis and affective neuroscience, and thereby also to illustrate what I mean when I say that the clinico-anatomical method is not the only method that can legitimately be described as neuropsychoanalytic. However, it must be said that some authorities distinguish between research in which psychoanalytic methods are applied directly and research in which psychoanalytic *theories* and *concepts* inform research (both human and animal) using other, more conventional neuroscientific methods. Katerina Fotopoulou calls the latter approach "psychodynamic neuroscience", which she distinguishes from neuropsychoanalysis proper (see Fotopoulou, 2012).

Part IV concerns a red thread that has run through the entire history of neuropsychoanalysis—namely, the attempt to empirically reconcile psychoanalytic and neurophysiological findings regarding dream theory. Whereas Parts II and III exemplified neuropsychoanalytic perspectives on neurological and psychiatric disorders, this section (and Part V—see below) exemplifies the neuropsychoanalytic perspective on normal mental functions. There are few such functions that have played so important a role in the development of psychoanalytic theory as has dreaming. This is why—given the bridge-building aims of neuropsychoanalysis—the topic of *The Dreaming Brain* (Hobson, 1988) was a special focus of neuropsychoanalysis from the start. The outcome of our efforts—namely, an almost complete vindication of Freudian dream theory after its vehement rejection in the 1970s and 1980s (see Hobson, 1988; Hobson & McCarley, 1977; McCarley & Hobson, 1977)—demonstrates the necessity of checking findings derived from animal models against those in human beings, who can describe their subjective states. For what are dreams if not subjective states? The outcome of our efforts in this area also demonstrates the importance of taking subjective states seriously—that is, of remembering that the mind is first and last a subject. Neurophysiologists like Alan Hobson based whole neuropsychological theories of dreaming on animal experiments in which it was quite impossible to monitor the actual dreams (as opposed to the objective states that *correlate* with them), but they made no attempt to check the *causal* basis of these correlations in humans—even though it was perfectly easy to do so. This fact can only be understood on the basis of pervasive prejudice against subjective states in contemporary neuroscience. As Semir Zeki put it: "most [neuroscientists] would shrink in horror at the thought of investigating what appears so impenetrable a problem" (1993, p. 343). And yet, as our findings showed, this prejudice led those neuroscientists very seriously astray.

I am confident that this section of the book will also illustrate the important role that neuropsychoanalysis has to play in defending hard-won psychoanalytic knowledge in an era when neurophysiological observations trump psychological ones no matter what, even to the point where scientists are driven to commit such basic methodological errors as to conflate correlation with causation. As I stated at the outset, neuropsychoanalysts do not believe that the mind can be reduced to the brain—that the mind can be eliminated from science—but that does not mean that the mainstream of contemporary neuroscience agrees. Bearing in mind that the mainstream has the ear of the general educated public, there is an important battle to be won here, and I believe neuropsychoanalysis has a major role to play in winning it.

For more technical accounts of the scientific findings underpinning neuropsychoanalytic dream theory, see Solms (1995, 1997a, 2000a, 2001b, 2011, 2012).

Part V serves to correct any misimpression perhaps created by the preceding section that the role of neuropsychoanalysis is to vindicate psychoanalytic theories—to prove that Freud was right all along. I have never subscribed to this view. Rather, I agree with the way that *Newsweek* science writer Fred Guterl once described our aim: "It's not a matter of proving Freud wrong or right, but of finishing the job" (2002, p. 51). It was absolutely inevitable when we began to systematically test Freud's theories against the sort of evidence that modern neuroscience provides that we would eventually learn that he was mistaken in some important respects. Freud himself predicted as much (recall his remark: "They may . . . blow away the whole artificial structure of our hypotheses"; 1920g, p. 60). But few people could have predicted, and certainly I myself never did, that we would be driven to overturn such a basic and cherished notion—almost an axiom—as the view that the id is unconscious. But that is exactly what we have been forced to conclude in the last few years.

The two publications that make up this section were both originally written for non-psychoanalytic (mainly neuroscientific and philosophical) audiences, but the arguments they contain are, I hope, set out in a way that should be accessible to most readers. In the case of the first of these (chapter 10) the general reader can simply ignore all the anatomical terms. The only important anatomical fact cited there that must be grasped in order to follow the argument is the distinction between the brainstem and the cortex, and this distinction is hardly an arcane one.

For psychoanalytic readers, I would like to emphasize the words I used to close another version of this chapter:

> Neuroscience is no more the final court of appeal for psychoanalysis than psychoanalysis is for neuroscience. The final court of appeal for psychoanalysts is the *clinical* situation. Readers are therefore invited to check the theoretical innovations I have introduced here against the data of their psychoanalytic experience. Do these new concepts really make better sense of the facts we observe? [Solms, 2013, p. 18]

The other publication in this section, chapter 11, takes these matters a little further and elaborates on the central philosophical theme of neuropsychoanalysis—namely, dual-aspect monism, first introduced in Part I. In doing so, this chapter applies our counter-intuitive findings regarding the "conscious id" to the search for the Holy Grail of contemporary neuroscience—namely, to what the philosopher David Chalmers (1995a, 1995b) calls the "hard problem" of consciousness. Philosophically minded readers may usefully supplement this chapter with my earlier treatments of the problem (Solms, 1997b, 2000b). (For psychoanalytically educated readers interested in my first stab at the clinical implications of these findings, see Solms, in press.)

One last remark before letting the reader loose: Please remember that the publications comprising this book were written at different points in the development of my work, and they are not presented in chronological order. Also, none of them should be treated as a definitive statement, either of my views or the views of neuropsychoanalysts as a whole. They are selected only from among my own publications, which cover a more limited range of topics than the total field of neuropsychoanalysis. They are also not representative of my own work, nor are they my "best" (or favourite) publications. My aim when making this selection was merely to provide the general reader with a digestible number of publications, written in a sufficiently accessible format, that cover an adequate variety of neuropsychoanalytic topics, to illustrate what I, at least, think this field is about.

PART I

WHAT IS
A NEUROPSYCHOANALYTIC
PERSPECTIVE?

CHAPTER ONE

What is neuropsychoanalysis?

Mark Solms & Oliver H. Turnbull

The first formal use of the term "neuro-psychoanalysis" occurred in 1999, when it was introduced as the title of the journal by that name. Plainly, however, the relationship between psychoanalysis and neuroscience is much older than the term. In the dozen years since the word "neuropsychoanalysis" was first used, it has been employed in a number of different ways, for different purposes, by different people.[1] This chapter serves to briefly survey some of this complexity and, in the process, to sketch out the intended scope of the field. In doing so, we will also address some of the criticisms that the field has encountered in the decade or so since its foundation.

There are two major limitations to this account. The first is that we can speak only for ourselves and thus describe what *we* think "neuropsychoanalysis" is—and ought to be. Nevertheless, we may

This chapter was first presented orally as Solms, M. (2009), "What is neuro-psychoanalysis?", at the 10th International Neuropsychoanalysis Congress: "Neuropsychoanalysis: Who needs it?", Paris. It was first published as Solms, M., & Turnbull, O. (2011), "What is neuropsychoanalysis?", in *Neuropsycho-analysis*, 13: 133–145.

claim a certain privilege in that respect, by virtue of one of us (MS) having invented the term. Second, we aim to speak only of the absolute basics of the discipline, to address only the foundational issues.

We will address the question "what is neuropsychoanalysis?" under four headings: (1) the historical foundations of neuropsychoanalysis, (2) its philosophical foundations, (3) its scientific foundations, and lastly (4) we will discuss what neuropsychoanalysis is *not*.

The historical foundations of neuropsychoanalysis

When we speak of the historical foundations of neuropsychoanalysis, we must of course begin with Freud. In doing so we are also addressing the question as to whether or not *neuro*psychoanalysis is really a legitimate part of psychoanalysis. The alternative view is that it is somehow a foreign body in our midst, or a deviation, or perhaps even something fundamentally *anti*-psychoanalytic.

In relation to this question, Freud's attitude to the issue is of paramount importance. If neuropsychoanalysis is legitimately part of what Freud conceived psychoanalysis to be, it places the inter-discipline of neuropsychoanalysis in a strong position with respect to this "parent" discipline. It was Freud, after all, who invented psychoanalysis. Happily, therefore, Freud's view on the matter was very clear, and also consistent throughout his life. Freud was, of course, a neuroscientist and a neurologist for the first two decades of his professional life (Solms, 2002; Solms & Saling, 1986; Sulloway, 1979). Throughout his later psychoanalytic work he had a specific scientific programme in mind, largely continuous with his earlier neuroscientific work, albeit shaped by the limitations of the scientific methods and techniques available to him at that time (for more on this topic see Solms & Saling, 1986; Solms, 1998a; Turnbull, 2001).

Freud's programme was to map the structure and functions of the human mind, and naturally he recognized that these were intimately related to the structure and functions of the human brain. However, as regards the mapping of these relationships, he consistently argued that the brain sciences of his time did not have the *tools*, in both conceptual and technical terms, necessary for exploring these relationships. He therefore shifted to a purely psychological method—a shift that he reluctantly saw as a necessary expedience. Just a few quotations illustrate this position:

> We must recollect that our provisional ideas in psychology will presumably some day be based on an organic substructure. . . . We are taking this probability into account in replacing the special chemical substances by special psychical forces. [Freud, 1914c, pp. 78–79]

> The deficiencies in our description would probably vanish if we were already in a position to replace the psychological terms by physiological or chemical ones. [Freud, 1920g, p. 60]

> Biology is truly a land of unlimited possibilities. We may expect it to give us the most surprising information and we cannot guess what answers it will return in a few dozen years to the questions we have put to it. [Freud, 1920g, p. 60]

There are many such statements throughout Freud's work. All reveal, first, that he viewed the separation of psychoanalysis from neuroscience as a *pragmatic* decision. Second, he was always at pains to clarify that progress in neuroscience would have the inevitable result that *at some time in the future* the neurosciences will advance sufficiently to make the gap bridgeable. As one of the quotes above suggests, his rough estimate was that this might happen in a "few dozen years". That was in 1920.

What were the methodological limitations that Freud encountered at that time? The main neuroscientific tool then available was the clinico-anatomical method, based on the clinical investigation of patients who had suffered focal brain lesions (Finger, 1994)—that is to say, studying how different functions of the mind were altered by damage to different parts of the brain. It was effectively the *only* method available for studying mind–brain relationships (though Freud's later years did briefly overlap with early developments in neurochemistry; see Finger, 1994).[2] However, Freud regarded the clinico-anatomical method as unsuitable for his purposes, despite having used it himself in his pre-analytic work. Best known is his 1891 book on the aphasias, which demonstrates how sophisticated was his mastery of that method, and of its limitations (for a modern appreciation of Freud's early neuropsychological investigations, see Shallice, 1988, pp. 245–247).

In that book, and in the papers that he published soon after (Solms, 2001b), Freud rejected the clinico-anatomical method, as he made the transition into psychoanalysis. He did so for several reasons. First, he recognized that the mind is a dynamic entity. It was Freud's emphatic view, even as a neurologist (Freud, 1891), that the mind was not made up of static modules or boxes connected up by arrows. Instead, Freud saw the mind as comprising dynamic, fluid processes. Second, Freud observed that the mind consisted in far more than consciousness; there was, beneath consciousness, a vast sub-structure, the workings of which had to be explored and understood before we would ever be able to make sense of the volitional brain.

The aim of psychoanalysis then became to develop a method and ultimately to derive from that method a theory (and a therapy), that would enable science to explore and understand the dynamic nature and unconscious structure of the mind. It is widely known that Freud then proceeded to use this purely clinical method, free from neuroscientific constraints, from 1895 or thereabouts, until 1939. This pioneering work left us a vast legacy, including a series of theoretical models of the basic organization of the mind, which we now refer to as "metapsychology".

Some psychoanalysts, misreading Freud, argue that the theoretical work of psychoanalysis must continue to remain aloof from neuroscience forever. We must avoid using neuroscientific methods, no matter how far these advance, and cling to our exclusively clinical, psychological approach. These are authors who question "whether the study of [neuroscience] contributes in any way to the understanding or development of psychoanalysis as theory or practice . . . whether neuroscience is of value to psychoanalysis *per se*" (Blass & Carmeli, 2007, p. 34; for a further opinion, see Karlsson, 2010, pp. 40–64). The proponents of this view appear (fortunately, in our opinion) to form a diminishing minority (British Psychoanalytical Society, 2008), but we must acknowledge that there are still some colleagues who believe that psychoanalysis has nothing to learn from neuroscience *in principle*. (Oddly, however, they do seem to think that neuroscience has something to learn from psychoanalysis!)

Independently of this theoretical—or ideological—question, there remains the *technical* question as to whether neuroscience has developed sufficiently as a discipline to allow it to make an adequate contribution to psychoanalytic theory: whether the methodological limitations (and related limitations of neuropsychological knowledge that Freud referred to) still remain. Stepping back, it is clear that there have been huge technical and methodological advances in the neurosciences over the last several decades. To offer but the briefest historical summary:

Electroencephalography (EEG) was introduced in the 1930s (Berger, 1929), though it was not fully exploited until after the war. This represented the beginning of a capability, initially rather crude, to measure and observe dynamic aspects of brain activity under changing functional conditions. The later development of event-related potentials (ERPs) in the 1960s (Sutton, Braren, Zubin & John, 1965; Sutton, Tueting, Zubin & John, 1967; Walter, Cooper, Aldridge, McCallum, & Winter, 1964; for a recent review see Luck, 2005) offered substantial advances over the basic EEG technique, by virtue of experimental control and averaging procedures. The recent development of magnetoencephalography (MEG) represents a further substantial advance, allowing us to study the neural dynamics associated with mental events at the millisecond level, with increasing anatomical precision.

In another domain, after the Second World War, there were tremendous developments in neuropsychology, using the lesion method in a new way which adapted its inherent limitations to the dynamic nature of the mind. Alexander Luria, in particular, developed a method known as "dynamic localisation" (Luria, 1966, 1973; see Kaplan-Solms & Solms, 2000, pp. 39–34; see also Solms & Turnbull, 2002, pp. 64–66). This method permitted the investigator to identify constellations of brain structures that interact to form functional systems, where each structure contributes an elementary component function to the complex psychological whole. On this basis, modern neuropsychology has a well-developed understanding of most of the basic mental functions. This applies especially to cognitive functions.

Further enormous technical advances followed the advent of computerized tomography in the 1970s, which made it possible to identify the precise location of a brain lesion while the patient was still alive. This was followed by magnetic resonance imaging (MRI). And from the 1990s onward, functional neuroimaging (functional magnetic resonance imaging, fMRI; positron emission tomography, PET; and single photon emission computed tomography, SPECT) made it possible to *directly observe* neurodynamic processes under changing psychological conditions.

It is now also possible to deliver temporary, short-acting "lesions" to neurologically intact research participants—either through sodium amytal injection (which was first introduced in the 1940s) or through magnetic pulses delivered to the outside of the skull via transcranial magnetic stimulation (TMS; which had been readily available since the 1990s). Innumerable other technologies also exist, ranging from stimulation of the cortical surface in neurosurgical operations (Penfield & Boldrey, 1937; Penfield & Rasmussen, 1950), through deep-brain stimulation (Mayberg et al., 2005), through psychopharmacological probes (Ostow, 1962, 1980), to mention only the most obvious examples.

Even this brief summary demonstrates that we *do* now have neuroscientific methods that enable us to study the dynamic nature of the mind and to identify the neural organization of its unconscious substructure. Each of these methods has its limitations, as all methods do, and there are undoubtedly many future advances to come—but the landscape of scientific enquiry in this domain has, certainly, *radically* changed since Freud's lifetime. For this reason, it seems entirely appropriate to reconsider whether we might now attempt to map the neurological basis of what we have learnt in psychoanalysis about the structure and functions of the mind, using neuroscientific methods available to us today. Freud would, in our opinion, have considered this a welcome and wholly legitimate development of the work that he pioneered. There has been something of an explosion in the number of books addressing this issue (e.g., Bazan, 2007; Bernstein, 2011; Corrigall & Wilkinson, 2003; Cozolino, 2002; Doidge, 2008; Fotopoulou, Pfaff, & Conway, 2012; Kaplan-Solms & Solms, 2000; Mancia, 2006; Northoff, 2011; Peled, 2008; Shevrin, Bond, Brakel, Hertel, & Williams, 1996; Solms & Turnbull, 2002).

The philosophical foundations of neuropsychoanalysis

If we are to correlate our psychoanalytic models of the mind with what we know about the structure and functions of the brain, we are immediately confronted with the philosophical problem of how mind and brain relate—with the "mind–body problem". This opens huge philosophical questions. Are we *reducing* the mind to the brain, are we *explaining away* the mind, or are we merely correlating mind and brain? And if we are merely correlating them, what is the causal basis of this apparently compulsory correlation? Is the relationship hierarchical, whereby psychoanalysis studies mere epiphenomena of the brain? Or is the mind *an emergent property* of the brain? (Chalmers, 1995a, 1995b, 1996; Churchland, 1986; Searle, 1980; for a basic review of these issues, see Solms, 1997a, or Solms & Turnbull, 2002, pp. 45–66).

It is, of course, terribly important in this field to be clear about one's conceptualization of the relationship between the mind and brain. We favour a conceptualization (shared by Freud) that we think neuropsychoanalysis as a whole may be based upon. This approach is typically labelled "dual-aspect monism" (see Solms, 1997a; Solms & Turnbull, 2002, pp. 56–58).

Freud says, very clearly in many places, that the actual nature of the mind is unconscious (for review see Solms, 1997a). He uses the phrase "the mind *in itself*" referring directly to the philosophy of Kant. For Kant, our subjective being, the thing we perceive when we look inwards, is not the mind *in itself*: the mind in itself cannot be perceived directly. We can only know the mind via our phenomenal consciousness, which provides an indirect and incomplete *representation* of the mental apparatus and it workings. The actual ontological nature of the mind is something epistemologically unknowable: it necessarily lies behind (and generates) conscious perception. We can, of course, *infer* its nature from our conscious observations and thereby "push back" the bounds of consciousness, which is what the psychoanalytic method seeks to do. Ultimately, however, we can never *directly* know the mind itself. We must therefore have recourse to abstractions, derived from inferences, and built into figurative models: metapsychology.

Similar epistemological limitations hold for the theoretical abstractions of other branches of psychology—to the extent that they too attempt to describe the inner workings of (any aspect of) the mind. Even highly developed theories such as, for example, dual-route reading models (Coltheart, Curtis, Atkins, & Haller, 1993), models of multiple memory systems (Schacter, 1996; Schacter, Norman, & Koutstaal, 1998), models of divergent visual systems engaged in perception and action (Milner & Goodale, 1993), and so on. *All* of psychology is ultimately just model-building of one sort or another. It is only the scale of Freud's metapsychology that distinguishes it, in this respect, from the more narrowly focused models of cognitive psychology and neuroscience. It is also (partly) for this reason that the metapsychology lacks some of the specificity of modern cognitive models. But that has no bearing on their ultimate epistemological limitations.

Freud argued not only that the mind is epistemologically unknowable, but also that it is ontologically no different from the rest of nature. Kant's view was that *everything* in the world as we know it, including the contents of our external awareness, is only an indirect representation of reality. What all scientists do is probe beyond this perceptual data to try to get a better picture of what Freud called the "the real state of affairs" (1940a [1938], p. 196). This approach, we note, is common to *all* the natural sciences— often with the use of artificial perceptual aids such as microscopes and telescopes and spectroscopy machines. They are ultimately all reduced to building *models* of our natural universe, and, in this way, the mind in itself exists on the same ontological plane as the rest of nature; it is just one of the things that we perceive.

It is unquestionably significant that evolutionary selective pressures advantage organisms that develop better—that is, more accurate—models of reality. In a world without vision, the first animals to evolve organs of sight would be highly advantaged. Those that develop *better* vision—for example, binocular viewing capabilities, a lens with adjustable focus, low-light detection capacities for twilight conditions, and so on—are further advantaged (for a readable account of the process, see Dawkins, 1998). And, so much more, those organisms that develop multiple sensory organs, each probing and sampling (and ultimately *representing*) a different aspect of the world around them. Considered across evolutionary time, organisms have, on this basis, developed successively better perceptually derived models of reality. Thus, the human mental apparatus (if functioning normally) delivers remarkably effective capabilities for perceptually guided locomotion, action, navigation, attentional selection, object identification, and object recognition. However, the fact that the perceptual systems offer only *representations* of the world can readily be demonstrated by the remarkable errors seen in visual illusions, as well as in psychotic hallucinations and dreams.

Freud argued that the model-building of physics is no different in principle from what we do in psychoanalysis—we begin with perceptions of our inner state, and then we make inferences about the true nature of the things that determine those perceptions. Our phenomenal consciousness gives us the *impression* that things are (from an external perspective) visual or auditory, or that things make us (from the internal perspective) sad or hungry, but these things are all merely *qualities* of consciousness. Our science, like all others, then strives to abstract "the real state of affairs" that lies behind them. Freud formalized all of this in his conception to the effect that consciousness has both internal and external "perceptual surfaces" (Solms, 1997a; Solms & Turnbull, 2002, pp. 18–31). The difference between psychoanalysis and the *physical* sciences is (on this account) merely the perceptual surface that we use.

Behind *both* of the perceptual surfaces lies something else ("reality itself"), which we can only build abstract models of. Forming better models of reality itself forms the goals of all science, including psychoanalytic science. It may surprise those who have forgotten the origins of psychoanalysis: for Freud his discipline was *always* a natural science, identical *in principle* with the other basic sciences, of physical reality, such as physics and chemistry. The mind in itself, then, is not ontologically different from—and not distinct from—the rest of the universe.

In sum, Freud was a monist, from 1900 all the way through to 1939. But his philosophical position can perhaps best be described as that of a dual-aspect monist (Solms & Turnbull, 2002, pp. 56–58), and so he was also a follower of Spinoza (cf. Damasio, 2004). Indeed, in Freud's correspondence he speaks highly of Spinoza (for an accessible survey see Damasio, 2004, p. 260), while in his published work he regularly described his position in Kantian terms (see Solms, 1997a, pp. 687–689).

If the mind, in itself, is unknowable, and we can only describe it with abstract models, such as Freud's model of the "mental apparatus", then we must take full advantage of the fact that our mental apparatus can be perceived in *two different ways*. If we look at it with our eyes (via the external perceptual surface), we see a *brain*: wet, gelatinous, lobular, and embedded within the other tissues of the body. If we observe it with our internally directed perceptual surface, introspectively, we observe mental states such as thirst and pleasure.

If we accept this philosophical approach, it follows naturally that we would want to make use of *both* points of view on our object of study, as perceived externally and internally. Why would we want to exclude, *a priori*, a full half of what we can learn about the part of nature that we are studying? In psychoanalysis, we adopt the viewpoint of subjectivity, because there are things that one can learn about the nature of the mental apparatus from this perspective, things that one can *never* see with one's eyes, no matter how much you aid them with scientific instruments. The philosophical position taken by some other scientists (for the opinions of Crick, Dennett, and Edelman, for example, see Solms, 1997a) *does* exclude this subjective perspective. Nevertheless, feelings exist; they are no less real than sights and sounds, they represent a fundamental part of the mind, and they can teach us a great deal about how it works. To exclude them *tout court* is actually crazy.

The information we can glean with our external sense organs, by studying the mental apparatus in its physical realization (the brain), is of course no less important. From a scientific point of view, there are actually a great many advantages that attach to studying physical objects. Some of our psychoanalytic colleagues (e.g., Blass & Carmeli, 2007; Karlsson, 2010) hold a contrary, exclusionary, position which we struggle to understand—not least because it seems irrational to deny oneself any source of useful data. Moreover, we should remind ourselves that the singular, fleeting, and fugitive nature of conscious states bestows distinct disadvantages; the more stable properties of the physical brain are more amenable to the requirements of the scientific method. Nevertheless, we reiterate that if one *correlates* the subjective experiences with the "wetware" of neurobiology, we are in a much stronger position to develop an accurate model of the mental apparatus itself. Thus, as with the moral of the blind men and the elephant, viewpoint-dependent errors are minimized. In sum, neuroscience offers a second perspective on the unknowable "thing" that we call the mental apparatus, the thing that Freud attempted to describe for the first time in his metapsychology.

Naturally, some in psychoanalysis have become anxious about how they might need to change their theories, and perhaps even their practice, by virtue of advances in knowledge that flow from such neuropsychoanalytic correlations.

Paradoxically, however, for us personally the interest has always been more in the *opposite* direction. In our early careers as neuroscientists, we became frustrated with how little we were able to learn about the essential nature of the mental apparatus and the lived life of the mind, with the cognitive neuroscience methods and theories that were available to us when we first trained (in the early 1980s). At that time (thankfully long past), neuroscience appeared to be blind to the fact that the brain was also a sentient being, capable of experiencing itself, with emotional feelings, volitional will, and a spontaneous sense of agency. The fact that these brain "mechanisms" are endogenously driven and motivated, that they arise out of the embodied nature of the subject, substantially affects the way the apparatus operates. These are not (we feel) epiphenomena, or details, or nice-to-haves: they are fundamental characteristics of how the brain works; they are what distinguishes the brain from the lung.

The scientific foundations of neuropsychoanalysis

The empirical basis for the discipline naturally flows from the facts described in the first section of this chapter, from the fact that Freud lacked confidence that the neuroscience of his time was capable of responding to the questions that psychoanalysis was putting to it.

We have argued (e.g., Solms & Turnbull, 2002, pp. 294–295) that subjectively experienced aspects of the mental apparatus are not, in and of themselves, an especially solid foundation on which to build a robust scientific discipline—given the fleeting and transient properties of subjective experience, the fact that (by definition) their phenomena can only be experienced by a single observer, and finally the fact that many aspects of mental life occur beyond subjective awareness. Surprisingly, even this apparently self-evident assertion has been challenged by our critics, who argue, for example that: "It would appear, according to Solms and Turnbull (2002, p. 46), that we have better access to atoms, molecules, quarks—that is, the non-perceivable perception of the world—than to our own subjective perceptual experiences." (Karlsson, 2010, p. 54). We concede that some aspects of nuclear physics and quantum mechanics may be difficult for the lay person to grasp, but the combined efforts of the scientific community, together with technical advances and the advantages of objectivity and observation replication, mean that physicists have a remarkable degree of precision in their understanding of the world—with mathematical formulae that predict physical properties (size, mass, etc.) to great accuracy. There is no aspect of subjectively experienced science which can begin to approach this level of precision.

Have there been advances in the neurosciences which might propel mental science towards the increased levels of understanding that is the goal of all science? Naturally the (mind–brain) problem is a more complex challenge than that which physics seeks to tackle. However, much has changed in the last few dozen years to move neuroscience in the correct direction. First, there were many technical and methodological advances in neuroscience (which we have already reviewed). These in turn led to genuine advances in our *understanding* of the mind and its workings, most notably flowing from the abandonment of radical behaviourism and the subsequent adoption of cognitive models by the psychological community. Thus, the last half-century has seen a dramatic advance in our understanding of (say) episodic memory (Scoville & Milner, 1957), visual attention (Posner, Cohen, & Rafal, 1982), executive control (Shallice, 1988), and visually guided action (Milner & Goodale, 1993), to mention but a few examples.

As we have suggested elsewhere (Turnbull & Solms, 2007, pp. 1083–1084), these findings in *cognitive* neuroscience have limited implications for psychoanalysis. Of potentially far greater importance are developments in the last two decades in the domain of *affective* neuroscience (Damasio, 1994, 1999b, 2011b; LeDoux, 1996, 2000; Panksepp, 1998a, 2011; Turnbull & Solms, 2007, pp. 1084–1085). Also very important have been significant advances in neuropsychology, the outstanding example being the discovery of "mirror neurons" (Gallese, Keysers, & Rizzolatti, 2004; Rizzolatti, Fadiga, Gallese, & Fogassi, 1996), as well as recent developments in social neuroscience (Cacioppo, Berntson, Sheridan, & McClintock, 2000; Cacioppo, Penny, Visser, & Pickett, 2005; Decety & Cacioppo, 2011). Finally, one should not overlook the many developments in psychoanalysis itself in the last century. Probably the most important of these is the line of "ethological" work on attachment, separation, and loss, running from Harlow (1958) through Winnicott (1960), Bowlby (1969), to Ainsworth (Ainsworth, Blehar, Waters, & Wall, 1978) and Fonagy and colleagues (e.g., Fonagy, Steele, & Steele, 1991; Fonagy & Target, 1996). An important conceptual turning point in our discipline was undoubtedly the publication of a pair of papers by Eric Kandel (1998, 1999) that offered a number of suggestions of research topics of relevance to neuropsychoanalysis, as well as providing much-needed support for the very idea of research in neuropsychoanalysis—an important badge of credibility for the field, especially as Kandel won the Nobel Prize (in 2000) for his work in medicine/physiology.

Importantly, however, individual developments in either of the "parent" disciplines of neuropsychoanalysis do not *themselves* bridge the divide between the fields. There have, however, been a number of bold attempts at such bridging, through the decades. The work of Paul Schilder (2007), Mortimer Ostow (1954, 1955; see also Turnbull, 2004) and Edwin Weinstein (Weinstein & Kahn, 1955) serve as beacons in this regard. Unfortunately, none of these earlier attempts flourished into the fully fledged interdiscipline we enjoy today, in part, perhaps, because each of these early attempts ran into the same difficulties (of means, motive, and opportunity) that Freud had encountered (for an interview with Ostow on this topic, see Turnbull, 2001).

In retrospect, one of the most central limitations may have been the lack of a significantly well-developed dynamic *neuropsychology*.

This only fully emerged in the 1970s, especially through the efforts of Luria (1966, 1973; for review see Kaplan-Solms & Solms, 2000, pp. 26–43, or Solms & Turnbull, 2002, pp. 25–27). The second transformational shift occurred with the full development of affective neuroscience in the 1990s (Damasio, 1994, 1999b; Panksepp, 1998a), which finally aligned neuroscience with the topics of fundamental interest to psychoanalysis, allowing the disciplines to share findings not merely in relation to cognition, but also in the core psychodynamic domains of emotion and instinctual drive. We will discuss this issue in more detail later in this chapter.

The bridging work that catalysed our own present interest in neuropsychoanalysis began in this context, with one of us (MS) doing relatively conventional psychoanalytic investigations of neurological patients (Kaplan-Solms & Solms, 2000). Why did this prove to be such a seminal approach for neuropsychoanalysis? First, it involved a clinical method that followed on directly from where Freud had left off. The method requires relatively modest changes in working practice, and little additional training on the part of a psychoanalyst, and yet gives direct access to the subjective mental life of the (neurological) patient in precisely the same way that psychoanalysts traditionally gather data about psychiatric (or "normal") patients.

This ensures that we can make direct observations concerning the neural correlates of metapsychological concepts in a methodologically valid setting. All of our metapsychological concepts and theories about the structure and functions of the mind are operationalized in a *clinical* psychoanalytic setting. Analytic work with neurological patients is therefore an ideal way of ensuring that we are studying the same "things" that Freud studied, albeit from a neurological perspective.

We would like to add a further reason why clinical work in neuropsychoanalysis is best performed with *neurological*, rather than *psychiatric*, patients. This is due to the methodological advantage of working with patients with *focal* brain lesions. First, most of these patients are pre-morbidly "typical" examples of humanity, with (as a population) few of the potentially confounding issues of aberrant development which often occur in psychiatric disorders (Bentall, 2003, 2009). Second, and most importantly, it enables us to correlate our psychoanalytic inferences with *definite* neuroscientific ones. Structural neurological lesions provide infinitely more precision than do psychopharmacological manipulations, considering all the interactive vagaries of neurotransmitter dynamics. Moreover, by virtue of advances in structural imaging, it is possible to identify the neural basis of the clinically observed phenomena in neurological patients with a high level of scientific accuracy—a method well-suited for establishing clinical-anatomical correlations (Heilman, & Valenstein, 1979; Kertesz, 1983; Kolb & Whishaw, 1990; Lesak, Howieson, & Loring, 2004).

In sum, having researched small populations of such patients (Kaplan-Solms & Solms, 2000), we have developed a method that offers a respectable degree of experimental control, a reasonable degree of neuroanatomical localization, excellent construct validity, and a direct observational window into the subjective life of the brain in a reasonably naturalistic setting.

On the basis of this approach, we have been able to build a preliminary picture of how our most basic metapsychological concepts might be correlated with brain anatomy and with all that we know of the functional organization of the brain. To take one example, in Kaplan-Solms and Solms (2000) we describe psycho-analytic observations on a small series of patients with right parietal lesions. They exhibited a remarkable degree of self-deception, in that they were paralysed (on the left side) but insisted that they were *not* paralysed. In some cases they explained away their paralysis through transparent rationalizations ("I tired the arm out this morning doing exercises"), or they developed more complex delusions—such as that the paralyzed arm belongs not to them but to the examiner, or to a close relative (for examples, see Aglioti, Smania, Manfredi, & Berlucchi, 1996; Feinberg, 2001; Ramachandran & Blakeslee, 1998). Cognitive neuroscientists have traditionally explained these remarkable clinical phenomena in terms of simple cognitive *deficits*—damage to inferred cognitive "modules" (for review, see Nardone, Ward, Fotopoulou & Turnbull, 2007; Turnbull, Jones & Reed-Screen, 2002; Turnbull, Owen & Evans, 2005). When we studied such patients psychoanalytically, however, we observed a pattern of psychological phenomena that was not at all modular in nature, and which was not by any means accurately defined as "deficit". What we observed were dynamic phenomena, in which the primary interacting forces clearly revolved around *emotional* states. Moreover, these emotionally determined dynamics caused important aspects of the cognitive processes involved to become *unconscious*. By intervening psychoanalytically in these dynamics, moreover, it was possible to reverse the dynamic process in question, and return the repressed cognitions to consciousness. This empirically demonstrated the validity of our conclusions, and it required students of this clinical phenomenon to radically reconceptualize its nature.

Kaplan-Solms and Solms (2000) concluded that self-deception in right parietal lobe damage might well be attributable to narcissistic defensive organizations, such that the patients avoided depressive affects, using a range of primitive defence mechanisms. This regression to narcissism appeared to be attributable to a loss of capacity for whole-object relationships (Kaplan-Solms & Solms, 2000, pp. 148–199). These patients also appeared to have disrupted cognitive processes that represent space correctly, as acquired through normal development. Of course, this begs the question of *why* the effect should be seen typically with right-sided legions. A likely explanation is that the sort of emotion-regulation systems that are mediated by the right convexity are lost in such patients, disrupting their ability to tolerate powerful negative affects (Fotopoulou, Conway, Solms, et al., 2008; Fotopoulou, Conway, Tyrer, et al., 2008; Fotopoulou, Solms, & Turnbull, 2004; Turnbull, Jones, & Reed-Screen, 2002; Turnbull, Owen, & Evans, 2005). These findings can be seen to confirm the relationship between realistic spatial representation (of self/object boundaries) and maturation of object relationships. It also pointed to the neural correlate of what in psychoanalysis is termed "whole-object" representation, the metapsychological foundation of mature object love.

However, while this approach of applying clinical psychoanalytic methods to the study of neurological patients has many strengths, it also has limitations. Because clinical observations necessarily involve limited experimental control, and are open to confirmation bias (Kahneman, 2003), it is a relatively weak method for determining the precise causal mechanisms involved.

Experimental studies, following on from those purely clinical observations, were therefore employed to provide fuller empirical support and refinement of the above hypotheses. A series of publications (Fotopoulou, Conway, Solms, et al., 2008; Fotopoulou, Conway, Tyrer, et al., 2008; Fotopoulou, Solms & Turnbull, 2004; Nardone et al., 2007; Tondowski, Kovacs, Morin, & Turnbull, 2007; Turnbull, Jones, & Reed-Screen, 2002; Turnbull, Owen, & Evans, 2005) have now conclusively demonstrated the powerful influence of emotions and unconscious cognitions (and associated defensive processes) in the neurodynamics that underpin the false beliefs of right parietal patients. For example, such patients show excessive attention to words that refer to paralysis and disabilities, despite *denying* that they are disabled and paralysed (Nardone et al., 2007).

These lines of work have been an important contribution to behavioural neurology, taking forward the ideas generated in neuropsychoanalysis beyond our own sphere or interest. As a result of these efforts, a psychoanalytic point of view is now included in conceptualizations of these phenomena in mainstream neuroscientific journals, and the influence and contribution of psychoanalysis to the neurosciences is spreading, apparently for the first time in history.

Simultaneously, psychoanalytic observations on how the mind is altered by damage to different parts of the brain has enabled us to begin to build up a coherent model of how the mental apparatus, as we understand it in psychoanalysis, is realized in anatomy and physiology, providing what we might call a new "physical" point of view in psychoanalytic metapsychology. We have made especially remarkable progress in this respect in relation to the psychoanalytic theory on dreams (Solms, 1997b, 2000, 2011) by using multiple converging methods. It has been gratifying indeed to rediscover the Freudian conception of dreams in the neurodynamics of the sleeping brain. So much so that in 2006, at the "Science of Consciousness" Conference in Tucson, Arizona, a formal Oxford-Rules debate (Solms vs Hobson) on the contemporary scientific validity of the Freudian conception of dreaming resulted in a 2-to-1 vote in our favour. While such renewed demonstrations of confidence in our most basic theoretical propositions may be regarded as merely sociological phenomena, they are not unimportant for the future viability of our discipline.

What neuropsychoanalysis is not

We have described what neuropsychoanalysis *is*—in terms of its historical foundations, philosophical premises, and empirical underpinnings. We turn now to what neuropsychoanalysis is *not*, by defining of some boundary conditions.

The first boundary is a methodological one. We have especially recommended the clinico-anatomical method of making *direct* psychoanalytic observations on patients with focal brain lesions, in a clinical setting. However, this is just a starting-point. We have pioneered an example of how such clinical observations can be extended, using experimental neuropsychological tools. We have already alluded to the multiple converging methods that were used to establish the neural organization of dream psychodynamics. But numerous other approaches are possible. Thus, to take a relatively extreme instance, one might manipulate different neuro-peptides in research participants who are *themselves* psychoanalysts, and then have them describe their subjective states, using their expertise in doing so (with reference to the theoretical concepts that we use). Approaches such as this are rather radical, but they have huge potential and appear to be remarkably under-appreciated. To take a less radical example, why do we not have systematic psycho-analytic studies of the manipulations of the different classical neu-rotransmitters that psychopharmacologists regularly tinker with in conventional psychiatric settings (cf. Kline, 1959; Ostow, 1962, 1980; Ostow & Kline, 1959)?

Other psychoanalytically informed neuroscience comes from the use of neuroimaging methods—for example, studying Freud's theory of mourning (Freed, Yanagihara, Hirsch, & Mann, 2009), psychodymanic aspects of confabulation (Fotopoulou, Conway, Solms, et al., 2008; Fotopoulou, Conway, Tyrer, et al., 2008; Foto-poulou, Solms, & Turnbull, 2004; Turnbull, Berry & Evans, 2004; Turnbull, Jenkins, & Rowley, 2004) or tests of Freud's dream theory (Solms, 1997b, 2000). We might wonder, of course, whether work of this sort can legitimately be called "neuropsychoanalysis", given that the data collection occurs using merely neuroscientific and psychological, rather than psychoanalytic, methods. Such work might best be described as *psychoanalytically informed neuroscience*. But who cares? On balance, we prefer to take the "broad church" approach to this issue—such that neuropsychoanalysis represents *all* work that lies along the psychoanalysis/neuroscience boundary; it may at times involve psychoanalytically inspired neuroscience (using purely neuroscientific methods to test psychoanalytically informed hypotheses), and at other times the direct psychoanalytic investigation of neurological variables (brain injury, pharmacological probes, deep-brain stimulation, etc.). What unites these approaches is that they are attempts to do neuropsychoanalytic *research*.

There is another way of doing "neuropsychoanalysis" that relies entirely on speculative imaginings, transpositions, and guesses. The classic instances of this arise from psychoanalysts reading something about the latest developments in the neurosciences and observing that the new findings are vaguely reminiscent of such and such phenomenon or theory in psychoanalysis. They then claim that this or that neuroscientific finding discloses the biological correlate or underpinning of some aspect of psychoanalytic theory. In our view, "armchair" speculation such as this does not represent the way forward for our field. The last century saw more than enough speculation in psychoanalysis, leading to the formation of multiple "schools of wisdom" but remarkably little scientific progress. There is only one way to decide between theories, and that is to *test* them against reality, in such a way that the alternative predictions can be either confirmed or disconfirmed. The "Project" (Freud, 1950 [1895]) was a notable early instance of such speculative guesswork, which is why Freud himself so strongly resisted its publication, describing it as an "aberration".

One further instance of what neuropsychoanalysis is *not* is worthy of mention. Neuropsychoanalysis is not (in our opinion) a "school" of psychoanalysis, in the way that we currently speak of Freudian, Kleinian, Intersubjective, and Self Psychology schools. Neuropsychoanalysis, we feel, is far better conceptualized as a link between *all* of psychoanalysis and the neurosciences. Alternatively, it might be described as an attempt to insert psychoanalysis into the neurosciences, as a member of the family of neurosciences—the one that studies the mental apparatus from the *subjective* point of view.

Finally, we would like to make it clear that neuropsychoanalysis (or neuroscience in general) is not a final "court of appeal" for psychoanalysis. Psychoanalysis cannot look to any other science to find out what errors it may have made in its methods, theory, and practice. This is not to say that neuroscience brings no information to bear on what may have been erroneous or misleading paths in psychoanalysis. We have been criticized, in the past (Karlsson, 2010, pp. 50–51) for not offering concrete instances of such errone-ous paths.

Thus, to take one powerful example, there is abundant evidence in neurobiology for the existence of what we refer to as "drives" (Panksepp, 1998a; Pfaff, 1999; Rolls, 1999). For some students of psychoanalysis, drive theory has been rejected as outmoded and inappropriate (Kohut, 2009; Siegel, 1996). Do recent neuroscientific observations invalidate this conclusion in psychoanalysis? They may not, but they are highly relevant to our ongoing thinking. It may be that the term "drive" is used in a quite different way by the psychoanalytic and neuroscientific communities (Fotopoulou. Pfaff, & Conway, 2012). Or it may be that the concept of drives is more relevant to some aspects of mental life than others. Or perhaps it may be that it is only the psychoanalytic *taxonomy* of the drives that needs revision. Other interpretations are also possible. Never-theless, it seems appropriate that the psychoanalytic community looks again at the data that led them to reject Freudian drive theory and investigates whether drives may play a more substantial part in mental life than they had previously thought.

Plainly, this is not the whole story; it is merely the beginning. Once we have started to ask ourselves these questions, based on our reading of the current state of drive theory in neurobiol-ogy, we must *test* their conclusions using our own, *psychoanalytic* techniques. This is bound to lead to new observations, not only of psychodynamic phenomena or continuities that we had not noticed before, but also of possible limitations or errors in the neurosci-entific conceptions at issue. It is, after all, more than possible that behavioural neuroscientists might have missed something impor-tant about the drives, deprived as they are of much of the data of subjective experience.

Thus, in our opinion, the interface between psychoanalysis and neuroscience is a rather *dialectical* one. As analysts, we may learn something new about the brain that seems relevant to psy-choanalysis. We may think about it, keep it at the back of our

minds, entertain the possibility, but above all *test it* psychoanalytically, as well as investigate its clinical usefulness. In this way, the
final court of appeal for psychoanalysis remains the psychoanalytic setting—psychoanalytic observations made on real human
beings, in the conventional clinical situation. A similar argument
might, in principle, apply to the neurosciences—though, of course,
they should and would never look to psychoanalysis as their
final court of appeal. The risk of reductionism seems always to
go in the direction of the physical, which is itself an interesting
neuropsychoanalytic phenomenon! But neuroscientists today *do*
look to psychoanalysis for interesting observations and theories,
which they are increasingly applying to their work. They also
quite naturally adopt them where they seem appropriate (Feinberg, 2001; Fotopoulou, Conway, Solms, et al., 2008; Fotopoulou,
Conway, Tyrer, et al., 2008; Fotopoulou, Solms, & Turnbull, 2004;
Ramachandran & Blakeslee, 1998; Turnbull, Berry, & Evans, 2004;
Turnbull, Jenkins, & Rowley, 2004; Turnbull, Jones, & Reed-Screen,
2002) and then move on.

The future

There is a long history in the sciences of remarkable creativity at
the boundaries between disciplines (Bowman & Turnbull, 2009;
Watson & Crick, 1953). Consistent with this, our interdisciplinary
field has already opened rich veins of new enquiry. Doubtless this
will continue to occur, and in unpredictable ways. Nevertheless we
would like to sketch a general outline that we would like the field
to move towards.

Our own vision is one of collaborative investigation of phenomena of common interest, approached using the rigour that is associated with all good scientific enquiry, but which also respects the
methodological tools (with all the advantages and disadvantages)
associated with each distinct field. An ideal outcome would be for
neuropsychoanalysis to avoid any suggestion of being an armchair
activity, or a field that is based on speculation rather than empirical work. Moreover, we envisage an inter-discipline in which the

acquisition of knowledge is bidirectional (psychoanalysis inform-
ing neuroscience, and *vice versa*), and a discipline that retains the
deep respect for the subjective perspective that is the hallmark of
psychoanalysis.

We are confident that this will be the outcome for our field—for,
as Freud told Einstein 83 years ago, "There is not greater, richer,
more mysterious subject, worthy of every effort of the human intellect, than the life of the mind" (Freud, 1929).

Note

1. There was a time when "depth neuropsychology" was the term used for
the new interdiscipline (Kaplan-Solms & Solms, 2000; Turnbull & Solms, 2003),
with reference to Freud's "depth psychology" (Freud, 1915e).

2. "The future may teach us to exercise a direct influence, by means of
particular chemical substances, on the amount of energy and their distribution
in the mental apparatus." (Freud, 1940a [1938], p. 182).

CHAPTER TWO

Putting the psyche into neuropsychology

Mark Solms

I trained in neuropsychology in the early 1980s. At that time (even more than today) the field was dominated by cognitive theory and methods. Accordingly, we learned a great deal about the manner in which the mechanisms of language, memory, visual recognition, and the like were organized in the brain, but we learned very little indeed about those aspects of mental life that were less readily amenable to computer-based models. Subjects like emotion, motivation, and personality were barely touched upon in my training in neuropsychology.

The great strength of scientific psychology in general, and neuropsychology in particular, is that it considers the mind objectively. The mind, is, after all, just a part of nature—it must somehow be reducible to lawful mechanisms that can be precisely defined in objective, third-person terms. All the achievements of scientific psychology derive from this. Especially in the case of neuropsychology, the fact that the mind can be literally objectified in the form of a physical organ is a great advantage. Studying mental mechanisms

---

This chapter was first published as Solms, M. (2006), "Putting the psyche into neuropsychology", in *The Psychologist*, 19: 538–539.

from the viewpoint of their physical basis in anatomy and physiology has enormous value from the natural–scientific standpoint, for it introduces into psychology all the possibilities of measurability and control that a physical science provides. The fleeting, fugitive stuff of the mind has always been an embarrassing handicap to scientifically minded psychologists. Neuropsychology changed all that—and that, no doubt, was part of its appeal for me, too, as I entered the field in the 1980s.

The problem with this approach, however, is the obvious fact that the mind is also *not* just another object. It is in the very essence of what we call "mind" that it is also a *subjective* thing. The mind could, in fact, perhaps best be defined as *the subjective aspect of nature*. When we say that the mind is just a part of nature, what we mean is that subjective experience—no less than other perceivable things—actually *exists*. We experience the world not only in the form of physical objects that we can see, hear, and touch, but also in the subjective form of feelings, volitions, and intentions. Such things, too, are therefore part of empirical reality. As such, they have causal, explanatory power. Much behaviour would be extremely difficult to understand without recourse to variables of this kind. Consider the case of suicide. How could one possibly explain the causal chain of events in a suicide without reference to emotional feelings and subjective thoughts—such as "my life is too painful to endure"? Although it might be possible in some absurdly roundabout way to exclude such things from our explanatory accounts, it would clearly require disingenuous re-labelling of a great deal of what actually happened. And what is the point of that?

I have always thought that what is most significant about the brain is the fact that it is not only an object. Unlike every other bodily organ it cannot be reduced to mechanisms alone, in the sense that it cannot be adequately described as *just* a machine. The defining characteristic, *the* distinguishing feature, of the brain is that—unlike the liver, lung, or stomach—it possesses subjectivity: that is, the capacity to *feel* what it is *like* to *be* a brain. Moreover, it has the capacity to *communicate* that feeling to other minds; the human brain can *speak* and *tell* us what it feels like to be what it is. These capacities provide us with an absolutely unique perspective on nature. And perhaps most important of all: the mind has *agency*. Unlike any machine, it is master of its own house, an intentional being in the world, possessed of that ineffable quality we call "free will".

Any science of the brain which ignores these facts will be ignoring the most essential distinguishing features of its object of study. And yet that was precisely what the neuropsychology of the 1980s seemed to want to do.

When I asked my professors about these things—about the neural basis of feeling, meaning, and the intentional self—I quickly learnt that one was not supposed to ask such questions in neuropsychology. I am sure I am not the only person who entered the field with the expectation that it concerned itself with exactly those things. If *psychology* is not concerned with them, then what science is?

I later realized (in analysis, as it happens) that I also had a more personal reason for wanting to understand these aspects of the brain. When I was 4 years old, my 6-year-old brother sustained a traumatic brain injury as a result of falling from a clubhouse roof while our parents were yachting. Needless to say, this dramatically altered the course of his life as well as the lives of all of us in the family. No doubt this event, and its painful sequelae, impressed upon me in a most direct way the real profundity of the link between mind and brain, between *person* and brain. It was, I am sure, the traumatic consequences that this connection caused my brother—more than any other single cause—that aroused my interest in the physical basis of the mind. And yet my teachers in the 1980s were telling me that things like personality and identity and self were not appropriate topics for a promising young student of neuropsychology to concern himself with. Such interests were, in fact, positively dangerous—at least as far as academic career prospects were concerned.

But still my frustrations at the limitations of the discipline grew. This was the origin of my interest in psychoanalysis. A friend in the philosophy department—of all things—suggested that I attend a seminar on Freud's "Project for a Scientific Psychology" (1950 [1895]). I remember well the mixed feelings I had in that seminar. It felt as if I were committing treason. But I quickly learned why I was there. Freud, for all his faults, was evidently a scientist of the kind that I aspired to be: he had clearly made a serious attempt to incorporate the mind (the real mind) into the realm of neurological science. He seemed to be a truth-loving researcher who, when confronted with the enormous difficulties implied by the very idea of a "science of subjectivity", decided that his methods had to be adapted to this subject matter, rather than the other way round. The other approach could only result in the exclusion of the human subject from science.

I was soon compulsively reading everything about Freud and his work that I could lay my hands on. To his enormous credit, my supervisor—while clearly disapproving—made no attempt to prevent me, while simultaneously making clear that nobody in neuropsychology at that time still took seriously the speculations that Freud laid out in his 1895 "Project", and even more so in his subsequent work.

I found it difficult to understand the prejudice. If Freud was wrong, or limited by the primitive scientific methods of his time, then surely all we needed to do now was subject his conclusions to modern scientific scrutiny. Using modern technology, such as neuroimaging, it would surely be possible to test, revise, and replace his findings where necessary. Surely that was preferable to excluding the *subject matter* of psychoanalysis from science.

My determination to take the former course was greatly strengthened by the knowledge that Freud himself had been a neuropsychologist. He had in fact made very valuable contributions to aphasiology, and had *introduced* the concept of agnosia in the early 1890s. He had only abandoned the study of the brain—very reluctantly—due to the lack of any valid methods for exploring the neural basis of the complex mental phenomena he discerned in his clinical work. This historical origin of psychoanalysis provided a useful foundation for re-integrating Freud's later contributions with neuropsychology. Freud was, after all, one of *us*: he *thought* like a neuropsychologist, at least in what came to be known as his "metapsychological" writings.

And so I decided to jump ship. In 1989 I began training in psychoanalysis at the Institute of Psychoanalysis in London. In the ensuing years I was gradually immersed in the methods and findings of that discipline—devoted to the study of real lived lives. Needless to say, there were once again many frustrations and disappointments along the way, but at least I was now among colleagues who were *trying* to understand the things that had interested me all along.

What was lacking, of course, was adequate scientific control, which was closely linked in my mind to the lack of any serious effort on the part of analysts to discover the *neural basis* of the complex mental processes that their clinical work had uncovered. This, then, was the contribution that I myself could make. Basing myself on the enormous advances that had occurred in neuropsychology in the intervening century, I could find the neural foundations that Freud had sought in vain. This could serve as a starting point for a new, deeper neuropsychology of the person. I immediately set out to research the brain mechanisms of dreaming, my rationale being that dreaming was the mental function that Freud (1900a) had chosen to use as the starting point for his first attempts to conceptualize the overall structure and function of the mind. If I could establish the neural correlates of *this* aspect of his model, I assumed, I would have forged something of a Rosetta Stone for correlating the findings of psychoanalysis with those of modern neuropsychology. The results of my efforts in this direction quickly paid dividends (Solms, 1995, 1997b, 2000). Thereafter, I broadened my focus in various directions, concentrating mainly on complex neuropsychiatric phenomena produced by focal brain injury, such as anosognosia and confabulation (Fotopoulou, Solms, & Turnbull, 2004; Kaplan-Solms & Solms, 2000; Solms, 2001a; Turnbull, Evans, & Owen, 2005).

The unfolding results of this exciting work have more than vindicated my decision to take psychoanalysis seriously. On this basis, I and a growing number of like-minded colleagues have established a new interdisciplinary area called "neuro-psychoanalysis", the simple aim of which is to introduce the psyche into neuropsychology—to demonstrate that the brain cannot possibly be understood if the subjective aspect of its nature is neglected or even ignored (see www.neuro-psa.org).

In closing, if I may be forgiven for quoting a journalist in this context, I can think of no better description of what neuropsychoanalysis aims to achieve than what Fred Guterl (2002) wrote in *Newsweek*: "It is not a matter of proving Freud wrong or right, but rather of finishing the job." I am delighted to be participating in that task.

CHAPTER THREE

What is the "mind"?
A neuropsychoanalytic approach

Mark Solms

I. Introduction

1. Since our engineering colleagues' ultimate aim seems to be the construction of an artificial mind—and since they wish to use our (neuropsychoanalytic) knowledge in this regard—it is an ideal opportunity to address the question I have framed in my title: what is a "mind"? In the process of addressing this question, I will of necessity also consider two related questions: where do minds occur in nature? (localization), and why do they exist? (function).

2. It is one thing to address such questions, and another to do so neuropsychoanalytically. What is special about the neuropsycho-

---

This chapter was first presented orally as Solms, M. (2007), "What is the mind?", at the 1st International Engineering & Neuro-Psychoanalysis Forum, Vienna; and it was presented again in many other forums thereafter in substantially different versions. It was first published as Solms, M. (2007), "What is the 'mind'? A neuro-psychoanalytical approach", in the *Conference Proceedings: 1st International Engineering and Neuro-Psychoanalysis Forum*, pp. 21–24; it was republished in a slightly revised version as Solms, M. (2008), "What is the 'mind'? A neuro-psychoanalytical approach", in D. Dietrich, G. Fodor, G. Zucker, & D. Bruckner (Eds.), *Simulating the Mind: A Technical Neuropsychoanalytical Approach* (Vienna: Springer), pp. 115–122.

analytic approach to this question? The engineering colleagues to whom I am responding (Dietrich, Fodor, Kastner, & Ulieru, 2007) enthusiastically adopt the psychoanalytic approach, but they do not tell us why they have turned specifically to this approach to the mind.

3. Freud (1923a [1922]) says that the psychoanalytic approach consists in three things: it is a therapy for treating mental disorders, a theory about the mind and its workings, and a method for investigating those workings.

4. Most people (Dietrich et al. included) seem to think of psychoanalysis mainly as a theory. There are in fact, especially nowadays, many different theories that are called "psychoanalytic". To call a theory "psychoanalytic" therefore begs the question. Dietrich et al. (who have no reason to bother themselves with such matters) implicitly answer the question by limiting themselves to Freud's psychoanalytic theory. But Freud frequently reminded us that scientific theories are of necessity provisional things—they are always subject to revision. The problem therefore remains: what about Freud's theory cannot be revised if it is to still qualify as "psychoanalytic"? What is enduringly psychoanalytic about a theory?

5. Many people know that psychoanalysis is a special form of therapy (the "talking cure"). But this aspect of psychoanalysis is no less subject to revision than its theory. Indeed, the therapeutic technique of psychoanalysis is largely derived from, and only makes sense in relation to, its theory.

6. This aspect of psychoanalysis is perhaps least relevant in the present context; our engineering colleagues want to construct an efficient mind, not to fix a broken one. I will therefore not discuss the mechanisms of psychopathology and techniques of psychotherapy here. I will only say in passing that, to the extent that the engineers succeed in accurately emulating the human mind, to that extent they will find that their model is prone to certain types of malfunctioning. One is almost tempted to use this as a criterion of their success!

7. Psychoanalysis is least well known (and perhaps least well respected) as a method of scientific enquiry. However, in my opinion, this is the most fundamental aspect of psychoanalysis—its most enduring and most unique feature. The psychoanalytic method

consists essentially in a certain mode of listening to the (ideally unedited) introspective observations of a person concerning his/her current mental experiences.

8. The raw data produced by such introspective reports provides information about the mind that cannot be obtained in any other way. Such data (derived from subjective observation) represents nothing less than half of what can be known about the mind (the other half being derived from objective observation—observation of the brain and behaviour).

9. The last-mentioned conjunction makes it possible to have such a thing as neuropsychoanalysis.

II. Subjectivity

10. The mind is unique in this respect: it is the only part of nature that can be known directly—that is, subjectively. Apparently the mind alone knows what it feels like to be itself. Moreover, in the case of the human mind, it can provide a verbal report about this subjective state of being. This is the rationale for the psychoanalytic method.

11. It is surely not a matter of indifference that the mind has this unique property. The use and investigation of this property is likely to reveal something of fundamental importance about the mind—something that exposes how and why it differs from all other biological things (indeed, from all other things in general). It will therefore be of considerable importance, in relation to the question we have set ourselves ("what is the mind?"), to review what we in psychoanalysis have discovered about this unique property: subjectivity.

III. The unconscious

12. Before doing so, however, I must point out that the psychoanalytic method consists in more than merely gathering introspective

reports. That would be phenomenology. What sets psychoanalysis apart from phenomenology is not just the nuanced complexities of psychoanalytic listening (evenly suspended attention, free association, empathy, transference, countertransference, interpretation, and the like) but, rather, a presupposition that underpins all these technicalities.

13. It is important to recognize that this fundamental feature of psychoanalysis does indeed boil down to a presupposition—and one that blurs the distinction between psychoanalytic method and psychoanalytic theory. Although this presupposition can be justified both empirically and logically (Freud, 1915e), it is nevertheless also true that it literally creates the domain of psychoanalytic enquiry.

14. In psychoanalysis we presuppose that the events that occur in the gaps and discontinuities in introspective experience (e.g., the events that cause unbidden thoughts or memories to occur, as if from nowhere) deserve no less than the continuous, conscious remainder to be described as "mental". This is the starting point of all psychoanalytic enquiry: the inference that a large portion of what we call the "mind" is unconscious. This conceptual innovation creates a universe of natural phenomena (a complete chain of causes and effects) that can be studied scientifically like any other aspect of nature. Without this presupposition, subjective experience cannot be studied scientifically. It (or at least a good portion of it) would always have to be translated into some other ontological plane, outside the mental sphere—probably into something neurological. With that, the notion of a "mental" science would effectively disappear.

15. The possibility of a purely mental science is thus created by the psychoanalytic method, the technical peculiarities of which are aimed at inferring the missing (unconscious) mental events that best explain the observed discontinuities in subjective experience. The missing material is thus translated into the language of experience ("interpretation").

16. What is essentially psychoanalytic therefore is the attempt to systematically study, understand, and influence the part of nature that we call "mind" in purely mental ways.

17. There is a complication relating to this fundamental feature of psychoanalysis that I hesitate to introduce, but it cannot be avoided. It is this: we do not believe that the mind is mental in itself (in Kant's sense). We believe that the subjective universe created by the above-described fundamental proposition is an observational perspective on the mind, not the mind itself. Subjectivity (the introspective perspective) is mere perception. The mind itself is the thing represented by introspective perception.

18. Saying that the unique feature of the mind is subjectivity (10 above), and then saying that subjectivity is mere perception of the mind (17 above), leads to confusion. But this apparent confusion is only semantic and will be rectified (21 below).

19. The philosophical complication just introduced is not a unique feature of subjectivity (introspective perception); it applies equally to objective perception. Perceptions, whether inwardly or outwardly derived, are always representations of something. What distinguishes inward (subjective) from outward (objective) perception is certain empirical features, first discovered by Freud, the most important of which is this:

20. Inward perception encounters resistances. These resistances are intimately bound up with the emotional feelings encountered by inward perception. (Emotional feelings are a unique feature of subjectivity; see 40 below.) In general, subjects want to avoid things that generate unpleasure (this is Freud's "pleasure principle"). When mental things that generate unpleasure cannot be avoided, the subject's primary tendency is to misrepresent them (this is the "primary process"). Facing unpleasant internal facts requires special mental effort (this is the "reality principle", governed by the "secondary process", to be described below).

IV. Different meanings of "mind"

21. Returning now to where we left off (11 above): what is the "mind" or the "mental"? To answer this question, we make a semantic distinction. In neuropsychoanalysis we distinguish between three grades:

22. mental *experience* (which is subjectively perceived—and provides the singular data of psychoanalytic enquiry);

23. the *organ* of the mind (the brain—which is objectively perceived, and provides the data for the various neurosciences);[1]

24. the mental *apparatus* (which is an abstraction—a model—a virtual thing, and is inferred from the two above-mentioned empirical sources).

25. The possibility of using the second set of data to correct viewpoint-dependent errors derived from the first set (and vice-versa) is the fundamental rationale for the existence of neuropsychoanalysis. This is because the aspect of nature—the "thing" in Kant's sense—that both psychoanalysis and neuroscience try to understand is the mental apparatus.

26. I am not saying anything too controversial, I hope, if I assert that mental experience (22) is what most people mean by "mind". This concomitant of the brain (23) is what sets it apart from all other organs of the body (and all other natural things).

V. Basic features of the mind

27. What, then, does mental experience consist in? It seems to involve three basic (but overlapping) features:

28. It is conscious. When the mind is not conscious it literally disappears as a mind. (This might seem to contradict point 14 above; but unconscious subjective events do not exist as such—as actual, empirically observed phenomena. They exist only as inferences—as hypothetical mental events. They therefore have the same ontological status as the "mental apparatus"—point 24)

29. It is intentional. Mental experience is always about something, always directed toward something. (Freud speaks here of "wish".)

30. It has agency (or free will). The experiencing mind makes decisions by and for itself: "I shall do this." (Even though the actual degrees of freedom are limited by the "reality principle", the experiencing mind always retains potential for radical freedom—as

is demonstrated by certain forms of insanity which disavow the reality principle.)

31. We shall see below that these three basic features of mental experience are intrinsically linked.

32. The brain possesses none of the above-mentioned special features. It is simply a bodily organ, no different in principle from the heart or the liver. Put differently, when the brain is considered from the subjective perspective (when it is considered from the perspective of consciousness, intentionality, and agency) it is no longer called the "brain", it is called the "mind".

33. These conclusions do not bode well for Dietrich et al.'s project. How does one begin to construct a machine with these features? Subjectivity is the very antithesis of machinery.

VI. A model of the mental apparatus

34. I can only suggest that we approach the problem from an indirect perspective. If the "mental apparatus" (24) represents the set of laws we have derived about the mind and its workings from the two sets of empirical data represented by 22 and 23 above, and if it alone unites them (as they must be united, since they are perceptions of the same underlying thing), then the "mental apparatus" should not be despised as something beyond reality. The mental apparatus is the mind itself—in Kant's absolute sense. Mental experience is mere appearance—mere perception—whereas the things we infer from the study of experience (and of the brain) are the ultimate stuff of the mind. Such ultimate things are always abstracted, unobservable in themselves (like "gravity" and "electricity" and "quarks"). The mind in itself, like all ultimate things, can only be modelled; it cannot be observed directly.

35. What, then, are the functional principles governing the mental apparatus, insofar as we have been able to abstract them from psychoanalytic (subjective) observation? This is a functional question, but the anatomical point of view should not be ignored (cf. "localization"; point 1) and still less contradicted (point 25).

36. The localization of the mental apparatus suggests that its main function is to mediate between the endogenous needs of the organism (the internal milieu) and the external objects of those needs (the environment). In psychoanalysis we call the pressure exerted on the mind by endogenous needs "drives". It is the most basic "fact of life" that organisms cannot meet their needs (cannot satisfy their drives) autochthonously. If an organism is to stay alive and reproduce, which are the two essential things that an organism must do, then it needs to find, interact with, consume, copulate with, etc., things other than itself (with "objects" from the viewpoint of the subject). This is why life is difficult, why it requires work.

To this end:

37. The mental apparatus receives information from two great sources: from the outside world and from the internal milieu. This information-receiving function is called "perception". The first function of the mind (flowing from point 36) is to bring these two things together. This confluence is being in the world, which may be divided into elementary units: "I am experiencing this." In such units, "I am" is the product of internal perception and ". . . experiencing this" is the product of external perception.2

38. The mind registers traces of previous perceptual confluences of this kind (previous units of experience) and, by sequencing them chronologically, it also registers cause-and-effect sequences of events. This is the function of "memory", which greatly extends the function of perception—and renders cognition possible.

39. Memory, and the cognition derived from it, extends perceptual being in the world. This extended being is the "ego". However, the immature ego has little control over the information that flows through it. The control that is normally equated with "ego" (or agency) depends upon another function not yet described (see 48 below). The immature ego is at the mercy of its drives and the environment and only gradually acquires its agency.

40. Perceptions, memories, and cognitions acquire meaning not only by being ordered chronologically but also by being rated on a scale of biological value. This is the primary function of "emotion". Biologically successful confluences of drives and objects feel good (pleasure) and unsuccessful ones feel bad (unpleasure). This

is their meaning.3 In this way, quantitative events acquire quality. "Biologically successful" here means "advancing the cause of staying alive to reproduce" (cf. point 36) which is felt as satisfying.4

41. The values just described, much elaborated through development (memory and consequently cognition), will later form the bedrock of ethical sentiment.

42. This capacity to feel on the pleasure–unpleasure series is the biological purpose of consciousness. "Consciousness" is the most essential feature of any feeling and is inherently evaluative. Consciousness extends outwards from its subjective sources (evaluation of drive states) onto the external world (perceptions of objects): "I feel like this about that." Here we recognize the "aboutness"—or intentionality—referred to above (cf. point 29). This links two of the basic features of mental experience: consciousness and intentionality. All that remains is agency.

43. Attaching meaning to units of experience (40) generates a simple motivational principle. Motivation consists in desire to repeat previous experiences of satisfaction (and to avoid previous experiences of frustration). This is the function of "wishing", derived from the "pleasure principle", both already mentioned. The wishes of the immature ego possess compulsive force.

44. Motivation filters the present through the past in order for the subject to reach decisions about what is to be done. The decisions of the immature ego are more-or-less obligatory, they are essentially dictated by its wishes (see 39).

45. Decisions trigger actions, via the (motor) output channel of the mind.

46. Experience (memory) shows that actions can be satisfying in the short term but still biologically unsuccessful in the long term. This requires the development of a capacity to tolerate unpleasure in the short term—the capacity to take a long-term view. This capacity for delay we equate with "maturity". It depends on inhibition of action.

47. Inhibition of action permits "thinking". Thinking is inhibited (imaginary) action, which permits evaluation of potential (imaginary) outcomes, notwithstanding current (actual) feelings. This function we call "secondary process".

48. Secondary-process inhibition replaces compulsive, instinctual or stereotyped actions with considered ones. Considered action is the essence of agency. It implies ownership of action. Agency depends on inhibition. Free will, ironically, turns on the capacity to not act.

VII. Conclusion

49. This, in barest outline, is the functional plan of the mental apparatus—according to the findings of psychoanalytic research. Neuropsychoanalytic research, which recently began to sketch in broad brushstrokes the anatomical and physiological correlates of this living apparatus (Solms, 1996), and to correct the viewpoint-dependent errors of psychoanalysis (Solms, 2006), should be able to greatly assist Dietrich et al. in their ambitious quest to design an artificial equivalent.

Notes

1. *Behaviour* (the output of the brain) is likewise objectively perceived, and belongs in the same category.

2. The "I am . . ." statement referred to here relies upon a capacity for reflexive thinking, which depends on other functions not yet described (see note 3 and point 47 below).

3. "Pleasurable" versus "unpleasurable" does not exhaust the range of meanings. The various "basic emotions", which recognize certain primal situations of universal significance, arose during mammalian evolution from elaborations of the function described here (see Panksepp, 1998a). *Language* is a further elaboration of this primitive meaning-making function.

4. A pleasure-generating mechanism, once it exists, can of course be exploited independently of its original biological purpose. Herein lies the source of many psychological ills and social evils—but these do not concern us here.

PART II

NEUROPSYCHOANALYTIC
PERSPECTIVES ON
SOME NEUROLOGICAL DISORDERS

CHAPTER FOUR

Is the brain more real than the mind?

Mark Solms

Introduction

This chapter reflects on the place of psychoanalytic thinking in a scientific context in which mental illness is increasingly being reduced to physiological and chemical factors. A small series of neurological patients with severe emotional disturbances is presented, in order to demonstrate that emotional symptoms can be neither described nor explained in physical terms. Even in cases where an organic aetiology is indisputable, physiological factors can only be invoked to explain somatic symptoms and the physiological correlates of mental symptoms. The mental symptoms themselves can only be understood psychologically.

This chapter was first presented orally as Solms, M. (1994). "Is the brain more real than the mind?", at a Conference of the Association for Psychoanalytic Psychotherapy in the NHS: "Chromosomes on the couch: Addressing biological issues in psychiatry", London; and it was presented again in many other forums thereafter. It was first published as Solms, M. (1995), "Is the brain more real than the mind?", in *Psychoanalytic Psychotherapy*, 9: 107–120; it was republished in a slightly revised version as Solms, M. (2004), "Is the brain more real than the mind?", in A. Casement (Ed.), *Who Owns Psychoanalysis?* (London: Karnac), pp. 323–342.

There can be no doubt that mental phenomena are somehow related to physical and chemical processes. The mental effects of drinking alcohol (as opposed to water) suffice to prove the point. Yet, psychotherapists get uncomfortable when they are asked to consider the relationship between the mental phenomena they deal with in their patients and the physical processes occurring in their brains. To think about their patients in this way seems somehow inhuman, and to miss the most essential point of what they are doing. It is as if the very foundations upon which they base their way of thinking about and helping their patients has been brought into question. Behind the question—what is the relationship between the mental phenomena that you deal with in your patients, and the physical processes occurring in their brains?—psychotherapists detect an implicit challenge. This challenge is based on the assumption that the brain is "more real" than the mind.

Of course there are other ways of conceptualizing the relationship between the brain and the mind, but within contemporary psychiatry the assumption that the brain is "more real" is increasingly taking hold. Enormous inroads have been made in pharmacological treatments, not only of the psychoses, but more recently also of the neuroses, and even of ordinary unhappiness. Patients whom we always thought of as having nothing at all wrong with their brains are increasingly being described by our colleagues in biological psychiatry as suffering from neurochemical imbalances. We think of these patients as having personal difficulties, which we situate in their feelings and memories, but our biologically oriented colleagues think of them as having chemical disorders, which they situate in their brains and their genes. We have a comprehensive, internally coherent way of understanding and treating these patients that has nothing to do with their brains, and we are therefore confronted by a yawning chasm when we try to reconcile this perspective with our own.

There are still some patients who, we all seem to agree, have difficulties that are situated either in their minds or in their brains. But the contradictions inherent in dividing the clinical population up in this way is revealed by the very existence of a transitional group, who seem to have difficulties that can be conceptualized and treated in two completely different ways. Thus the relationship between the brain and the mind has ceased to be merely an interesting philosophical problem for us; it has become a matter of urgent and practical concern. In psychiatry today, strange as it may seem, the boundaries of the brain are being extended, and the mind is getting progressively smaller.

In this chapter, I am not going to approach these issues from a philosophical point of view. Philosophers themselves admit that the mind–body problem (in the way that they conceive of it) can never be resolved. Instead I will consider the problem in the light of some pertinent clinical material, to see if our psychoanalytic way of thinking about these cases can be reduced to processes occurring in their brains. Although I cannot be comprehensive, I hope that this clinical material will provide a useful basis for at least beginning to address these problems.

Clinical material

I will describe five patients (some of whom were treated by my wife and colleague, Karen Kaplan-Solms).

Mrs A

This 61-year-old retired nurse was referred from the neurosurgical wards of a large teaching hospital because she was profoundly depressed, following a stroke. She was constantly in tears and had twice tried to commit suicide, first by throwing herself down a flight of stairs and then by attempting to jump from a third-floor window. The only reason that she did not succeed in the second attempt was because she suffered from such dense hemiplegia, unilateral neglect, and spatial disorientation that she was unable to negotiate the window.

She had suffered a ruptured aneurysm in the right middle cerebral artery of her brain. The symptoms that she had as a result of her stroke were typical of right-hemisphere cases. The term "left hemiplegia" refers to a spastic paralysis of the left arm and leg, which confined Mrs A to a wheelchair. The term "unilateral neglect" refers to a strange symptom that is quite commonly seen in these cases: they completely ignore everything that they see or hear or feel on the left-hand side of space, even though there is nothing wrong with their senses of vision, hearing, and touch. They seem literally to "forget" that the left-hand side of space, and of their own bodies, ever existed. It sometimes happens with these cases that, if you show them their own left arm, they will actually deny that it belongs to them, and they will make this assertion with a sense of conviction that you cannot shake, no matter how much logical argument or factual evidence you marshal to contradict it. (The symptom of neglect sometimes takes on a different form—one could say, a paradoxical form— whereby the patient, rather than ignore or deny the existence of the left-hand side of the body, becomes completely *obsessed* by it.) The third symptom with which Mrs A presented was spatial disorientation, which is a self-explanatory term, and which is also a common consequence of damage to this part of the brain.

The symptom that caused her to be referred to our service, how- ever, is very unusual in right-hemisphere cases. I am referring to her depression. It is a well-established clinical fact, that whereas left-hemisphere cases are quite frequently depressed, and present with what is called "catastrophic reactions", right-hemisphere cases usually display a striking indifference to their symptoms, often actually denying that they are ill at all. They will insist, for example, that they are perfectly capable of walking (or run- ning) despite the obvious fact that they are in a wheelchair and that they cannot even stand. This symptom—which is called "anosognosia"—is closely related to the symptom of neglect. But Mrs A did not suffer from the usual form of anosognosia. She was extremely depressed, and it was for this reasons that we arranged daily sessions for her, in a psychoanalytic setting, to see if we could understand why she felt that she must kill herself, and thereby to see if we could help her.

In the very first minutes of her first session, Mrs A stated that the reason why she was in tears all the time, and feeling suicidal, was because "I keep losing things" and because "everybody hates me". These two thoughts, "I keep losing things" and "everybody hates me" ultimately revealed the basic structure of her depres- sion. This was because, first, her depression was a reaction to loss and, second, it was the product of a self-directed hatred. Mrs A herself explained, reasonably enough, that she was depressed and felt suicidal because, as a result of her stroke, she had lost her independence. Curiously, however, she was not fully aware of the equally obvious fact that she had lost the use of the left-hand side of her body. We are thus faced with a paradoxical situation in which Mrs A was depressed because she had "lost her independence", although she was simultaneously unaware of the essential cause of that lost independence—namely, her dense hemiplegia. This loss, which was the immediate cause of her depression, could only be expressed indirectly, by means of association with other losses, of which she *was* consciously aware, such as the death of her father decades before, an early hysterectomy, and the frequent losses of trivial objects—which resulted from her spatial disorientation and neglect—during her daily life in hospital. (This is what she was *consciously* referring to when she complained that she kept losing things.) This paradoxical situation, of being depressed about a paralysis of which she was unaware, provided a clue as to what had happened to her neglected body-half; a short period of analytic work revealed that she was not consciously aware of having lost her left arm and leg, because *she had denied the loss by means of an introjection*. Thus, the left side of her body was both there and not there at the same time. She neglected her real hemiparetic arm and leg because in her mind she still had them safely inside her. However, because her attachment to her own body had necessarily been a narcissistic one, her attitude towards these introjected lost objects was decidedly ambivalent. She understandably felt terribly let down by the left side of her body, upon which she—like all of us—had always depended absolutely, without ever realizing it. This part of her own beloved self, which she had naturally assumed was under her omnipotent control, had suddenly revealed itself to be a piece of external reality after all—and, moreover, it had revealed itself to be an unreliable piece of reality, an object that she needed and loved, but that had nevertheless abandoned her. Her constant refrain that "everybody hates me" therefore turned out to be a projection of an internal situation in which a previously healthy and independent part of herself was hated by a now-crippled and dependent part of herself.

Her hatred of this introjected image of her lost self could be traced back analytically to its infantile origins in her identification with her mother—that is, it could be traced back to her identification with the woman upon whom she had depended for so long during childhood. The earliest bond to the mother is always a partly narcissistic one, just as the attachment to one's own body is. As Freud (1923b, p. 25) has pointed out, the body as an object has a special status; it is simultaneously a part of the ego and a part of external reality. At least one analyst (Laufer, 1982) has demonstrated convincingly in this regard, especially in relation to masturbation, that our own bodies—and particularly our hands—unconsciously represent both our own selves and the physical care that we received from our mothers. Mrs A's internally directed hatred was thus directed not only towards an introjected image of her lost, fully functioning body; it was ultimately directed also towards her internalized mother, who was narcissistically and ambivalently cathected, and who was an object of absolute dependence, before she let the patient down so terribly.

In this we recognize precisely the configuration that Freud (1917e [1915]) described in his classical paper "Mourning and Melancholia". An ambivalently loved, narcissistically cathected object is lost, but the loss is denied by means of an introjection of that object; the lost object is thus preserved within the unconscious part of the ego, but it is simultaneously attacked with the ruthless vengefulness of a lover scorned. Thus the self-hatred of the melancholic is revealed to be the internal expression of a repressed hatred towards an external object, whose independent existence was never fully recognized in the first place, before it was lost.

Mrs B & Mr C

Now I would like to describe two somewhat different patients. These two patients, like Mrs A, both suffered strokes in the right hemisphere of their brains—one as a result of a haemorrhage and the other as a result of a thrombosis, also in the distribution of the right middle cerebral artery. They were both middle-aged professionals.

Like Mrs A, these two patients were both densely hemiplegic, and they both suffered unilateral neglect and spatial disorientation. However, unlike Mrs A, neither of these patients was depressed. Despite the fact that they suffered exactly the same physical defects as Mrs A, and had damage to precisely the same part of the brain, these patients were indifferent to their symptoms; in the case of Mr C, he actually denied that there was anything wrong with him at all. In other words, these two patients, rather than presenting with depression, presented with varying degrees of anosognosia.

What impressed the therapist was how narcissistic they were. They were impenetrable, detached, aloof, and superior—and although they consciously deplored the idea of being in any way dependent, they were demanding and complaining in a child-like way. Mr C was also rather hypochondriacal in regard to a variety of bodily processes—which created a strange contrast with his near-total denial of his dense hemiplegia. As is so often the case in the non-neurological population, the narcissistic veneer of these two patients turned out to be a rather brittle defence. Their pervasive "indifference" was only apparent. A small amount of psychotherapeutic work revealed an underlying sense of loss, and a profound fear of the humiliation and dependency it involved. These patients, no less than Mrs A, were unconsciously very much aware of the narcissistic blow they had endured, and of how vulnerable they now really were. Consciously, they denied any concern about the loss of status and independence which their physical incapacities implied, but unconsciously these things were very deeply felt. They were constantly on the brink of feeling completely crushed, and *the potential for depression, which this unconscious knowledge brought with it, was constantly threatening to overwhelm them.* This was easy to demonstrate analytically, as appropriate interpretations brought forth floods of tears and an all-consuming sense of loss, with regard to humiliations and failures about which they had apparently been blithely unconcerned just moments before. In these two cases, therefore, no less than in the first case, there was (to use Freud's felicitous phrase) an "open wound" in their narcissism (Freud, 1917e [1915], p. 253)—there was a gaping hole in the body image, through which the entire narcissistic supply threatened to drain. Their defence against this intolerable situation—if we think about it in terms of Freud's classical theory—was an introversion of object libido back upon the ego. In this way, the anosognosic denial of reality was applied like a patch over the wound in their narcissism. In other words, the ego was—as we say—hypercathected at the expense of reality and was thereby artificially reinflated. Just as Mrs A had defended herself against conscious awareness of the rent in her ego by means of an introjection of the lost part of herself, so Mrs B and Mr C defended themselves against this same situation by means of an equally narcissistic introversion, which took the form of an all pervasive denial.

On the basis of these findings, we may conclude that anosognosia can be understood as part of the general tendency in us all to repudiate a breach of our bodily integrity. However, that does not explain why patients with damage to the *right* side of the brain present with this symptom, while patients with damage to the left side of the brain do not, although they suffer an equivalent breach to their bodily integrity (and in fact a greater loss, since in most of them it is the dominant, right arm that is paralysed). I will return to this question a little later.

Before I do so, I would like to briefly describe a third group of right-hemisphere patients. These were two young men who, like Mrs A, sustained damage to the right hemisphere of the brain as a result of a ruptured middle cerebral artery aneurysm.

Mr D and Mr E

These patients, unlike the previous three cases, were consciously obsessed by their paralysed limbs. This is the paradoxical form of the neglect syndrome, which I mentioned to you earlier. Again, we studied these patients in a psychoanalytic setting.

These two patients, like the other three, were basically narcissistic, but in a different sense of the word. They were in an agitated and aggressive state, constantly blaming the medical and rehabilitation staff for causing their symptoms. Interestingly, both of them demanded that we make good this injustice by amputating

the offending limb. They were impatient, imperious, and obsessive; they were hyperactive, and they were intolerant of imper-
fection, frustration, and doubt of any kind. The notion that they
might obtain partial improvement through the slow process and
physical effort of a rehabilitation programme was anathema to
them. They wanted their bodies to be restored completely to
the *status quo ante*, or they did not want them at all. If we could
not fix the paralysed arm immediately and perfectly, then we
should, rather, cut it off and replace it with a prosthesis. Even if
that meant that they would be left with only the pincer movements of an artificial claw, it would be preferable to the disgust-
ing, malfunctioning appendage that was currently attached to
them. Their constant threat to us was that if we did not do as
they instructed, they would do it themselves, or kill themselves,
or even kill us. Their unconscious attitude seemed to be: "If
you do not give me the breast right now, immediately—exactly
when, where, and how I want it—then I will bite my tongue and
my mouth, and I will bite the breast, and I will spit out all the
pieces, and *that* will teach you a lesson." In fact, Mr E almost
said as much when he exploded in one session, saying that he
was going to bite his left hand to bits, and spit out all the pieces,
and then post them in an envelope to the surgeon who had
operated on him. There was no conscious recognition of the fact
that the reason why the surgeon had operated on him in the first
place was because the patient had been *born* with a life-threatening arterial abnormality that had now ruptured. The idea that
the source of his handicap lay within himself was intolerable; it
was the surgeon who had deformed him, and unless he fixed it
right now, he would kill himself, or the surgeon, or both. It is
important to note, moreover, that in the case I am describing the
hemiparesis was actually milder than it was in any of the other
four cases—it took the form of an occasional clonus (involuntary
twitching) of the left hand. But this clonus meant that the hand
had a life of its own, that it would not do the patient's bidding,
that it was no longer under his omnipotent control—and for this
reason it *had to be removed.* While he was making these threats,
the patient restlessly paced up and down the room, which is
something that he frequently did, in order to "let off steam", as
he called it.

I hope that this description reveals what the mechanism of the mental disorder was in these two cases. In the first three patients, the hand that had let them down (which straddled the border between the ego and the outside world, and which was therefore unconsciously equated with the ambivalently cathected, earliest mother-figure) was introjected into the ego, where it was violently attacked. However, in these two patients the hand was projected outwards, into the hated external reality to which it now so obviously belonged. To these patients, it was intolerable that the hand should remain a part of themselves, because if it did, they would be in the painful situation of the first group of patients—that is, they would have to hate their own beloved selves rather than reality—and that was a positively life-threatening situation. Thus, we can see that in these patients, too, the defence was ultimately directed against the possibility of depression.

I think it can be seen that the patients in the latter group were also distinctly paranoid. For as long as the bad object was perceived as being separate from them, they were constantly under threat from that quarter. In fact, we had a third case of this type at our hospital, who was *extremely* paranoid (and masturbated compulsively). However, it was not possible for us to investigate him analytically because he was acutely ill, and we had to become involved with the practical management.

Now, considering all of these patients together, we can understand how it happens that the same lesion can give rise to such apparently opposite syndromes. Indifferent neglect of a limb and agitated obsession with it are, in fact, two ways of expressing the same psychological conflict; the two syndromes share the same underlying dynamics, but they give rise to different defensive solutions. What all these cases have in common is that damage to a part of the normally functioning body was experienced as a profound narcissistic injury, which was associated with a deep and inseparable sense of loss, accompanied by an awareness of dependency upon the object. But this intolerable situation was avoided, by means of a narcissistic defensive process that involved a withdrawal of cathexis from the external object back into the ego, which was then split, either by means of introjection or by projection, together with an all-pervasive denial. In this sense, all cases with right-hemisphere damage that we have so far studied may be said to present with *a failure of the process of mourning.*

Discussion

In all the above cases there was a demonstrable and unambiguous lesion of the brain. That is why I have chosen to present neurologi-cal cases rather than psychiatric ones. If it can be agreed that the emotional symptoms in these cases were correlated with definite abnormalities of the brain, then we can throw into sharper relief the specific issue being considered; we can then separate it off from other controversial issues, such as whether we should consider a particular psychiatric disorder to have a neurochemical aetiology or not. In these five cases the matter was beyond dispute, and this allows us to concentrate upon the specific question regarding the nature of the relationship between the neuropathology and the psychopathology. I hope it is evident that despite the presence of a demonstrable lesion in these five cases, and despite the obvious aetiological role of the brain lesions, we still cannot reduce the psychological symptoms to the organic lesions. I believe that this is true for the following reasons.

First, we could have studied these patients' brains for as long as we liked, by every conceivable method, but unless we actually interacted with them as people, we would never have known what had happened to them. We would never have known, for example, that Mrs A was depressed, that Mrs B and Mr C felt indifferent, and that Messrs D and E were obsessed in a very particular way. These emotional symptoms were the fundamental psychiatric facts in these cases. But depression, indifference, and obsessions can never be found in the brain, nor in any other part of the body. Feeling states can, quite simply, only be found in the mind. What I am saying is, of course, quite obvious, and nobody would seriously dispute it. Nevertheless I think that it is worth reminding ourselves that there are things in the world that cannot be seen or heard or touched, but that can still be perceived and known and that are therefore *real* all the same. Certain things can only be perceived subjectively. If we accept this truism, then we cannot come to any other conclusion than the following one: the mind has a reality of its own. There is both a physical and a psychic reality.

But this does not answer the original question. "Certainly", I hear someone say, "the mind is real—if that's what you wish to call it—but nobody is seriously disputing that; what we are saying is that the reality of the mind *depends* upon the reality of the brain. The mind is *produced* by the brain. Therefore the brain is *more* real than the mind. The states of conscious awareness to which you draw attention may be descriptively or phenomenologically irreducible, but they were *caused* by an event in the brain. If Mrs A had not suffered a stroke, she would not have been depressed; and the same applies to Mrs B's and Mr C's indifference, and to Messrs D's and E's obsessions." The question then seems to be, *why* did these patients experience what they did? Were their subjective symptoms caused by something that happened in their brains, or by something that happened in their minds? This question is more complicated than it seems. In attempting to answer it, I suggest that we be guided by an example from physical neurology.

If we wished to understand what caused Mrs A's *hemiplegia*, for example, we would do so in the following manner. We would begin with the medical history and a thorough clinical examination. This would lead us to formulate a hypothesis—based upon our previous experiences of similar cases, and upon the documented experiences of innumerable colleagues before us—as to what caused this particular hemiplegia. Our hypothesis would be that this hemiplegia was caused by a subarachnoid haemorrhage. We could not have guessed that by *looking* at the hemiplegia, but we could infer it from the clinical history. We could then test this hypothesis by conducting a series of radiological and laboratory investigations. Information derived from these tests, combined with the history and our examination of the patient, would lead us to conclude that the subarachnoid haemorrhage was caused by a constitutional arterial abnormality (known as a cerebral aneurysm) that had now ruptured. We know where in the brain to look for confirmation of this conclusion. The location of the aneurysm—together with the extent and location of the haemorrhage that it produced (and its sequelae)—would fully explain the hemiplegia. As to what caused the aneurysm, we would postulate an inherited disposition. As for the origin of that predisposition, we would infer a genetic variation, which ultimately reflects the laws of natural selection. Proceeding in this way, as you can see, we would be able to reconstruct the entire causal chain, which we describe as the "mechanism" of the symptom. This causal chain unfolds as an unbroken sequence of natural events, over definite physical structures.

But can this type of analysis reveal the mechanism of the *emotional* symptoms? Can these physical investigations and procedures clarify why Mrs A was depressed, for example, or why she felt that she had to kill herself? I believe not. When we investigated the psychological symptomatology in the five cases that I have described, we started from the assumption that the symptoms were real things, even though they were subjective experiences. This reflected the truism that I have discussed already. But if the very nature of a subjective experience renders it inaccessible to physical methods of observation and description, then why should its causal mechanism yield to such methods? A moment's reflection reveals the futility of seeking the cause of a suicidal melancholia (for example) in a CT scan. A scan (or an angiogram, or whatever) can only reveal the cause of the stroke. To say that she was depressed "because" of the stroke (i.e., because a part of her brain was not working) begs the question. That is why, in the cases reported above, it seemed natural for us to explore the immediate causal determinants of the patients' subjective experiences by means of a systematic examination of the psychic context out of which those experiences arose. That is, we sought explanations for the psychic symptoms by delving more deeply into the psychic facts. This seemed appropriate, despite our knowledge that something was wrong with their brains. Just as the neurologist sets about examining the bodies of these patients, so we set about examining their minds. And just as the neurologist pursued his/her examination beyond the immediate clinical data with the help of artificial aids such as angiograms and CT scans, so we pursued our investigations beyond the limits of the immediate (conscious) data with the help of artificial psychological aids.

What are these "artificial psychological aids"? They are nothing other than the well-known techniques of psychoanalysis, which enable us to overcome the emotional resistances that conceal a patient's innermost thoughts, and thereby to follow their causal sequence beyond the threshold of consciousness. These techniques are, of course, not easy to master, but they are the only techniques available for investigating the causation of the emotional processes that are of interest to us. The results that these techniques provide do not enjoy the same degree of scientific certainty as the results that are obtained by the neurologist, but we may console ourselves with the knowledge that the difficulty of our techniques, and the controversy surrounding our results, are inevitable consequences of the manner in which the mind is constructed. Unlike physical objects, subjective states of awareness are not sharply delimited things; they are transient and fugitive states, and they cannot be publicly scrutinized. To put it differently, they cannot be perceived via our *external* sensory organs. But this does not mean that they do not exist. For that reason we are able to study them, using appropriate methods.

So, what did the psychoanalytic method of investigation teach us about the causal mechanisms of the emotional symptoms in these cases? We started from the observation that the five patients— all of whom suffered lesions of roughly the same type, in roughly the same part of the brain—presented with radically different emotional symptoms.[1] Analytic investigation revealed that these different symptoms—which I am describing as *depression, indifference,* and *obsession* for short—were produced by three different defensive reactions to a unitary psychic trauma. These defensive reactions were (in varying combinations) *introjection, denial,* and *projection.* These reactions were triggered by a primary breach in the integrity of the bodily ego, which threatened to expose these patients to unbearable states of mental pain, associated with an awareness of loss and dependency. These affective links were traced back to earlier psychological traumata, and ultimately to a primal narcissistic catastrophe that was associated with the process of becoming separate ("weaning"). This established a full causal sequence of psychological events, analogous to the physical sequence that produced the hemiplegia.

We have therefore arrived at the viewpoint that in order to understand the mechanism of emotional symptoms in a case of neurological disease, it is necessary to take account of the whole personality of the patient, including the pre-morbid ego organization. This is not surprising. It simply reflects the fact that by the time that these patients fell ill, they had already been through a lifetime of experiences, and that these experiences were different in each case. It also reflects the probable fact that the patients were born with different psychological constitutions. A stroke therefore has different psychological implications for different patients, who have different resources available for dealing with them. However, no matter how we construe these factors, the essential conclusion remains: *the different psychological mechanisms in each case—and therefore the causal chain of psychological events—could only be understood psychologically.* In other words, in marked contrast to the impotence of physical methods of analysis, a psychological approach to the emotional symptoms readily revealed their mechanism.

But this still leaves out of account the specific relationship between the anatomical damage and the emotional symptoms. I have said that the emotional symptoms were attributable to narcissistic injury. But why should bodily-ego disturbances arising from lesions in the *right* cerebral hemisphere in particular, produce severe narcissistic injuries of the sort that we detected at the base of these symptoms? Clearly, the two causal domains described above are linked at this point, and that link calls for an explanation. We must therefore consider how the physiological and psychological mechanisms described above related to one another. This is, in a sense, the crux of the problem we are considering.

If damage to the right hemisphere of the brain necessarily results in a profound narcissistic injury of the type described above, then the implication is that the two causal chains are correlated in a highly specific way. In neurological science, this type of correlation is designated by the term "localization". Does this mean that the narcissistically cathected presentation that we call the "bodily ego" (and the introjections based upon it) can be located in the right cerebral hemisphere? As a matter of fact it does not. Just as a narcissistic injury can never be found inside a brain lesion, so a mental function can never be located within an anatomical structure. This is because psychic and physical reality are organized in completely different ways. The nature of the relationship between the two domains is defined by the laws of cerebral localization. In accordance with these laws, we know—for example—that the bodily ego (an elementary mental structure) has a highly complex neural realization. The neurological correlates of the bodily ego begin at the sensory–motor periphery; they include large parts of the spinal cord, all of the cranial nerves, and numerous modality-specific nuclei in the brainstem and diencephalon, in addition to the primary sensory-motor regions of the cerebral cortex, the secondary cortical zones adjacent to them, and much of the association cortex beyond. Each of these structures subserves a physiological function that contributes a different component element to the functional entity known as the bodily ego. They contribute these same elements to numerous other mental functions too. Thus, depending upon the site of the lesion, neurological disease in these different structures correlates with a wide variety of different changes in the mental representation of the body, together with various, simultaneous changes in other aspects of mental life. There is nothing surprising in this finding. Modern neuropsychology has demonstrated that the same principles apply quite generally to human mental functions. Simple mental functions have widely distributed physical correlates, and simple physical structures participate in a wide variety of mental functions. For this reason, mental functions can never be found *inside* neuroanatomical structures; they exist, as it were, *between* them. More importantly, each mental function consists of more than the sum of the component physiological parts that correlate with them. Even if the physiological correlates could somehow be captured and localized, they would still only be correlates of a process of thought; they would not suddenly become the thought itself. This is why mental functions can never be reduced to their physical correlates. Reducing a mental function to the physiological processes that correlate with them is like reducing a poem to the letters of the alphabet. Such reductions are possible in principle, but the object being studied evaporates in the process. Once again, this is a direct expression of the fact that mental and physical states represent two completely different aspects of reality, each irreducible to the other.[2]

Applying these principles to the material at hand, we have found that the right cerebral hemisphere contributes a particular component function to the complex functional system that is the physical correlate of a simple mental presentation known as the "bodily ego". I do not have space to provide a detailed description of this component function here. I can only mention the basic facts. There seems to be a special relationship between the right-hemisphere association cortex and the representation of "things", as opposed to "words". In this respect, the cerebral representation of the body as a "thing" is inextricably linked with the cerebral representation of other "things". Consequently, damage to the right hemisphere of the brain results in a collapse, not only of our conception of bodily space, but also of external objects and of concrete space in general. This reflects the genetic (developmental) link between the representation of the body and the representation of the object world. In this sense, the world develops out of the body. Damage to equivalent cortical tissue in the *left* cerebral hemisphere affects symbolic representations of the body, which are bound into a closed system of lexical and semantic connections. Damage to these parts of the brain impairs bodily representations only in so far as they are encoded within an abstract system of connections. This has various important consequences, depending upon the aspect of the process involved. But the concrete presentation of the body itself remains largely unaffected. Left-hemisphere patients do not "forget" that parts of the body ever existed. This enables them to make realistic adaptations to their physical symptoms, and to institute the necessary process of mourning. These are some of the essential reasons why damage to the left side of the brain does not result in the severe narcissistic reactions that accompany equivalent lesions in the right hemisphere. However, in left-hemisphere patients the symbolic functions that words provide are impaired.[3]

The point I am making is this. It would be wrong to infer from the clinical data I have presented that the representation of the "thing" to which we are more deeply attached than to any other thing in the world—namely, our own beloved selves—can simply be removed like a piece in a jigsaw puzzle from the right hemisphere of the brain. Even the primary trauma involves a complex, dynamic process. Thus, for example, it is impossible to suffer damage to the concrete representation of the bodily ego (the ego as a "thing") without this immediately affecting the representation of external objects and of space. Trauma to this aspect of the bodily ego results in a gross distortion of external objects, to a collapse of external space, and to a withdrawal of object cathexes. This in turn results in a regression from object-love to narcissism, and so on. These interrelationships reflect the fundamental fact that mental life is in its essence a dynamic process, which carries within itself the whole of its developmental history. Processes of this type can never be concretely located in the anatomical structures of the brain.

My general conclusion is this: if it is true that the essential nature and the causal mechanism of a psychological symptom can only be revealed by psychological means in cases where there has been recent physical damage to a specific part of the brain, then how much more that must be so if the physical correlate (or even the aetiological factor) is a neurochemical imbalance, which may or may not have existed for the whole of the patient's life. And if what has happened to a person—and what is happening to them—can only be properly understood by way of their psychic reality, even in cases where the material reality is beyond any reasonable doubt, then how much more that must be so when even the specialists cannot decide what the material reality is. And if we have to take account in neurological cases of the fact that mental processes of the sort that we deal with in psychoanalysis are in a constant state of flux (that they are endlessly organizing, re-organizing, and adapting themselves to changing circumstances, and that they not only do so in the present, but that they have also done so in myriad ways throughout the long process of development), then how much more that must be the case if there has not been physical damage to the brain; how much more it must be the case if the physical correlate (or even the aetiology) is a neurochemical imbalance, which is in itself a dynamic thing, and which may or may not have existed for the whole of the patient's life. In short, I think that these cases demonstrate, even in instances in which the aetiological factors are best described in physiological terms, that we would be making a serious mistake if we concluded that the associated mental illness itself can be described or understood from a physiological point of view.

These are the essential reasons why I believe that we can never replace a psychological science with a physical one. Of course, that does not meant that the two things are unrelated. But what it most certainly does mean is that *the mind is no less real than the brain*; for that reason, no matter what advances might be made in future in neurological science, it would be foolish to believe that we will ever explain the psychological reality of mental illness by means of anything other than psychology.

In reaching these conclusions, I am not saying anything new; I am simply repeating something that Freud—who was himself a neuroscientist—taught us more than 100 years ago, when he tried to understand the mental symptoms of *his* neurological patients. Given more space I could have described how Freud (1891) arrived at those views on the basis of the mental changes that he observed in cases with damage to the left hemisphere of the brain, and how those observations led him to conclude that psychic reality could never be reduced to material reality, and how that led to the birth of psychoanalysis, and what effect this viewpoint (which Freud first expressed in a famous neurological monograph) had upon subsequent developments in science.

We still do not know how all of the complicated psychological phenomena that we deal with in our consulting rooms are correlated with the material structures of the brain. But if we approach this problem afresh, on the basis of the principles that I have described—in a way that takes as its starting point the primacy and the reality of conscious mental life, and that accepts as given the mental nature of the unconscious processes which determine it—then I see no reason why we should not be able to answer these questions someday. In other words, we will only be able to achieve this goal if we integrate a fully psychological psychiatry into the field of neurobiology. I would like to suggest that if we study psychologically the emotional symptoms that arise from neurological pathology, which necessarily means that we attempt to understand neurological patients using psychoanalytic methods, then I can see no reason why we will not eventually be able to understand the essential changes that have taken place in their lives, and how those changes correlate with the changes that have occurred in their brains. If we do this slowly and carefully, and do not forget the basic principles upon which our discipline was built, then I feel sure that we will gradually be able to differentiate between what is fundamental in those changes, and what is secondary, and between what is generally true for the human mind as a whole, and what is idiosyncratic to the individual concerned. In this way we can build an understanding of how the knowledge that we have gained about the depths of the mind relates to knowledge that has been gained about the brain, without us having to sacrifice any of the valuable insights that the pioneers of our discipline have passed down to us.

And if we can do this with structural lesions, I see no reason why we cannot do the same with neurochemical imbalances—if and where they can be demonstrated. I believe that this is an appropriate basis for reconciling our psychoanalytic knowledge with recent advances in the neurological sciences.

In this chapter I have been able only to hint at how this way of approaching the problem actually works in practice, and I have been able to describe only a fragment of the sort of data that it generates, but I hope that I have nevertheless been able to convince readers of the principle that this is a worthwhile way to proceed. Finally, I hope that if any readers find themselves in a situation in future where a neurological patient is referred to them for psychotherapeutic help, that they will not turn away from the task in horror but, rather, that they will grasp the real scientific opportunity that it presents.

Notes

1. The different symptoms—which in some instances were diametric opposites—cannot be attributed to minor variations in the location and extent of the lesions. All of these patients had damage in the dorsolateral convexity of the right cerebral hemisphere, in the distribution of the middle cerebral artery. Everything that we know about the functional organization of this part of the brain contradicts the view that such major symptomatic differences were due to minor variations in the lesions. In neuropsychology we customarily classify all the manifestations of right-hemisphere convexity damage under a unitary nosological heading—namely, *the* "right-hemisphere syndrome".

2. In Freudian metapsychology, we say that consciousness has *two perceptual surfaces*, which represent an underlying reality ("unknowable" in itself) in two completely different ways. These are the terminal points of conscious perception, from which it is simply impossible to free ourselves. The dualistic conception of brain and mind (in the pre-psychoanalytic sense of the word) is abstracted from these two categories of consciousness; it is therefore determined by the basic structure of the mental apparatus.

3. Words protect us from things. In Freudian metapsychology we speak of "stimulus barriers", and of a process called "binding", which transforms overwhelming concrete realities into manageable "signals" of the same. Accordingly, left-hemisphere patients are frequently unable to use language to distance themselves emotionally from their loss. This produces a characteristic set of emotional symptoms, known as the "catastrophic reaction". (This function of words is also disturbed in certain forms of psychosis.)

CHAPTER FIVE

An example of neuropsychoanalytic research: Korsakoff's syndrome

Mark Solms

This is a very informal account of the research activities in which I am involved, illustrated by just one example. My main interest is the relationship between psychoanalysis and neuroscience. I am conducting various types of research at this interface. Rather than give an overview of the entire field, which would be very schematic and, I think, very boring, I shall focus on just one aspect, for reasons that I hope will become clear. This is possibly the most pertinent aspect of my research. I also hope by this example to convey an idea of the scope of the opportunities that exist for psychoanalysis today in this area.

This chapter was first presented orally as Solms, M. (2001), "An example of neuro-psychoanalytic research: Korsakoff's syndrome", at the 10th Annual Research Lecture of the British Psychoanalytical Society, School of Oriental & African Studies, London; and it was presented again in many other forums thereafter in substantially different versions. It was first published as Solms, M. (2001), "An example of neuro-psychoanalytic research: Korsakoff's syndrome", in the *Bulletin of the British Psychoanalytical Society*, 37 (5): 24–32; it was republished in a slightly revised version as Solms, M. (2002), "An example of neuro-psychoanalytic research: Korsakoff's syndrome", in *Journal of European Psychoanalysis*, 14: 133–145.

My starting point is the belief that psychoanalysts and neuroscientists, or at least what are nowadays known as cognitive neuroscientists (neuropsychologists and behavioural neurologists), are studying fundamentally the same thing. We in psychoanalysis are interested, just as they are, in the human mind: how it works and what the laws are that govern its functioning. If it is self-evidently true that we are both studying and trying to understand the same thing, the same piece of nature, albeit it from different viewpoints and using different methods, then it is absurd that we have so little to do with each other. Surely we should be collaborating, comparing notes, and sharing our findings with each other. It is from this starting point that I have become involved in my field of research, an example of which I shall report. Psychoanalysts will find much of what I say self-evident, analytically speaking. It is neuroscientists particularly whom I wish to address.

What we do in psychoanalysis is attempt to understand the functioning of the human mind from the vantage point of *being* a human mind—that is, from the vantage point of inner experience. Our perspective on the mind is the internal surface of consciousness, as Freud would have called it. We look inwards. We try to study our patients by encouraging them to look inwards, and from their free associations, which are their attempt to describe as honestly and accurately as they can what it is that they are experiencing during the minutes that they are lying on the couch. We make inferences, firstly, about those individual patients and what is going on inside their minds at that particular moment. From that, we make inferences about that person in general; what the structure of his/her personality is and the underlying structure of the difficulties for which he/she has come to analysis in the first place. From there, we make abstractions about how the human mind in general works. The "functional architecture of the mind", as cognitive neuroscientists would describe it, is ultimately what we are trying to learn about.

Neuroscientists start from the vantage point of external perception, of looking outwards, observing the mind as it is realized as a physical organ, a thing, an external object. They try by various methods and approaches to discern what the functional architecture of the mind is. Thus, when neuroscientists describe a model of how memory works (and memory is central to the example I am going to be discussing) they are talking about exactly the same thing that we psychoanalysts are interested in, to the extent that we have a theory of memory and how it works.

Psychoanalysis rests largely on a single method of investigation: the clinical method. The methods of neuroscience are more various. Yet there is a method that, historically, had the same significance for cognitive neuroscience as our clinical method in psychoanalysis. This is the method of clinico-anatomical correlation. It was formally introduced into neuroscience in 1861 by Broca and it was championed by Charcot. Charcot, of course, had a great influence on Freud. The method involves making clinical observations about mental changes in a neurological patient, which follow from disease or damage to a particular part of the brain. The clinical observations as to how the patient's mind has changed are then correlated with anatomic observations—that is, with the site of the lesion (the damaged part of the brain). This correlation teaches us something about what the mental functions were of the part of the brain now damaged. This method of study is, as I said, not the only method in cognitive neuroscience. It has since been supplemented by numerous other methods. Yet, as I will show, this method is the obvious place for psychoanalysts to link up with the neurosciences if we are going to construct bridges across our two fields.

Starting in 1861 with this approach of trying to understand how the mind is altered by damage to different parts of the brain, neuroscientists have been able to develop a highly elaborated picture of the functional architecture of the mind, of how the mind works. These attempts to infer normal function from clinical observations and the anatomical location of lesions that produced them have traditionally, and of necessity, been *theory-driven*. One does not make clinical observations about the mind without a theory with which to organize those observations and guide one, whether as a neuroscientist or psychoanalyst. Broca began in 1861 with the theories of faculty psychology, which were fashionable at the time. These theories were rapidly replaced in behavioural neuroscience by the theories of association psychology. The theories of association psychology are not that far removed from those that guide the clinico- anatomical correlation approach to mental science today—that is, cognitive psychology. Behavioural neuroscientists today use a cognitive model to guide their exploration of the functional architecture of the mind. That model has served them well in their attempts to understand cognition, but, not surprisingly, it began to falter as neuroscience began to mature beyond the merely cognitive.

Neuropsychology has begun in very recent years to grapple with something that it previously excluded: the problems of personality, complex emotions, and motivation, the truly interesting aspects of psychology. This provides a unique opportunity for psychoanalysis to build a bridge to neuroscience, because psychoanalysis has a highly elaborated theory about these very aspects of mental life, which neuroscience is now starting to grapple with. Fortunately I am not alone in believing that psychoanalytic theories might be of particular help to neuroscientists who are beginning to tackle these complex problems of human subjectivity. I can align myself in this respect with a recent winner of the Nobel Prize in Medicine, Eric Kandel, who stated in an article entitled "A New Intellectual Framework for Psychiatry" (1998; see also Kandel, 1999) that this is the future of cognitive neuroscience. In order to grapple with this aspect of mental life, cognitive neuroscientists need to make a bridge to psychoanalysis, which still offers, in Kandel's words, "the most coherent and intellectually satisfying view" of personality, motivation and complex emotion (p. 505). Therefore, a window of opportunity exists here, and I for one am keen to climb through that window and make use of this opportunity. There are enormous advantages not only for neuroscience, but for psychoanalysis too. If we can find links between our psychoanalytically derived concepts on how the mind works and the concepts of neuroscience, then we can open our theory to an entirely new range of methodological possibilities, a new range of methods for testing hypotheses that we had previously been content only to generate. The psychoanalytic method is very useful for generating hypotheses about how the mind works and for making inferences, but psychoanalysts have historically not been very good at testing their hypotheses. There is a limit beyond which the psychoanalytic method cannot go, and this applies especially to deciding between competing hypotheses in a reliable, scientific way. By making links to the neurosciences, we create the possibility of testing some of our hypotheses in ways that might make it possible to move forward in what Freud called our metapsychology, our general theory of how the mind works. That is one of the obvious advantages for psychoanalysis of making these links. There is much more I could say about these general points, but I want to get to the main focus of this chapter.

My wife, Karen Kaplan-Solms, is my primary collaborator in using the method that I am going to describe, but, happily, we are being joined increasingly by more than a handful of colleagues. I should also state at the outset that we are very much aware that these are the very first steps. We are drawing very broad brush-strokes—the ABC's of trying to make anatomical or physiological descriptions of our basic psychoanalytic concepts. There is a great deal more that needs to be done beyond this first step, but the method that we use in trying to make these links is in fact not radically different from the clinico-anatomical method that I described a moment ago. We study patients with damage to circumscribed parts of their brains, just as Broca did and cognitive neuroscientists have done ever since. We try to understand how their minds are altered by the changes in their brains. However, the method that we use to make our clinical observations and the theory that we use to organize those observations are *psychoanalytic*. We study these patients psychoanalytically in order to be able to understand psychoanalytically how their personalities and their emotional and motivational life have been altered by the brain lesion. This gives us an initial rough sketch of how these aspects of mental life, as we understand them in psychoanalysis, might be represented in the tissues of the brain. So, it is basically the clinico-anatomical method that we use, the good old-fashioned "meat-and-veg" clinical method of behavioural neuroscience. The only difference is the nature of the clinical observations. Cognitive neuropsychologists use psychometric testing to elucidate the cognitive changes. This method is really not adequate for capturing the subjective aspects of mental life. In contrast, we try to capture the changes in these patients' minds by studying them and describing them psychoanalytically. We have used this method with a wide range of different lesions, and this is necessarily how one has to proceed. We study patients with damage to various parts of the brain, trying to group them together by anatomical region. For example, we researched a group of patients with damage to the right-hemisphere convexity. We studied the anosognosia-neglect syndrome, which emerges with damage to that part of the brain, and which results in some very interesting personality changes. I believe that, by looking at these patients psychoanalytically, we did in fact learn some interesting things (I reported on our findings with this group of patients at one of the British Psychoanalytical Society's Research Seminars; see Solms, 1999).

I am now going to illustrate the same method but by looking at a different region of the brain. The syndrome that I am going to discuss psychoanalytically by way of an illustrative example is *Korsakoff's syndrome*. This is a very bizarre, very disturbing alteration of personality that occurs when there are lesions in a particular area. The part of the brain that I am referring to is just in front of the third ventricle. There is some controversy about precisely what nuclei have to be involved in order to produce this syndrome. The dorsal medial thalamus seems to be an important focus in the production of the clinical syndrome. Lower down, the hypothalamus and the mammillary bodies are also important anatomical structures involved. The basal forebrain nuclei in the frontal lobe, and at least some tissue of the frontal cortex itself, are also increasingly believed to be implicated. The relevant areas are thus the dorsal medial thalamus, hypothalamus, basal forebrain nuclei, and frontal cortex.

One needs to bear in mind that the clinical picture I am going to describe is not what "brain damage" (in general) looks like; this is what brain damage looks like only when the damage is in this particular part of the brain. Obviously, if the damage is in a different part of the brain, a radically different personality change would result. Moreover, Korsakoff's syndrome is not to be confused with Korsakoff's disease. That is a disease entity, which was described along with Korsakoff's original description of this syndrome in 1887. A second paper on the disorder appeared in 1889. The earlier paper elucidated a particular disease process, essentially a vitamin deficiency, a result of chronic alcoholism, which affects this part of the brain. It was, however, subsequently realized that any disease process that affects this part of the brain produces the same syndrome.

The patient I am going to describe did not have Korsakoff's disease, he had a different disease, but it caused him to suffer from Korsakoff's syndrome. He is one of a group of patients described in more detail in a book written by my wife and myself (Kaplan-Solms & Solms, 2000). What I am about to discuss is the clinical syndrome, Korsakoff's syndrome, which occurs with damage to this part of the brain regardless of what the cause of the damage was or what the pathological process was. One of the other patients described in our book (Case G, p. 215) had an anterior communicating artery aneurysm, which is a kind of haemorrhage in that area. Another (Case H, p. 207) had a self-inflicted bullet wound in that area.

I am going to focus on a patient (not reported in our book) whom I saw recently in London. He had a tumour, a meningioma, in the aforementioned area of the brain, which was surgically removed. After the surgery, he woke up with this syndrome.

Korsakoff's syndrome has two main features. The first is amnesia. These patients have a profound loss of memory. According to the classical descriptions, they cannot lay down new memories. Thus, they might meet you at one o'clock today; you might walk out of the room and come back in at five-past-one and they won't know you. They will believe that they have never met you. What I am describing is not some esoteric rarity; it is quite common. This is the core feature of the syndrome. These patients are literally unable to lay down new memories. They live from minute to minute without having any recollection of what happened in the moment that has just past. This amnesia affects primarily the most recent events, especially those that occur after the onset of the disease. It does, however, also affect the older memories, but progressively less so, so that we have a temporal gradient: the further back one goes in time, the more secure the memories are. The more recent the memories are, the more unreliable (or non-existent) they are.

The second core feature of the syndrome, which distinguishes it from other amnesic syndromes, is that of confabulation. Rather than simply forgetting memories, rather than simply saying, "I don't remember", if, for example, one puts a direct question to them in relation to a memory test, these patients invent memories. They make up stories. They have false beliefs. They fabricate events. The technical term for all of these distortions is "confabulation". So these cases have not only a loss of memory but also a replacement of the gaps in their memory, as it were, by these florid inventions, which create the impression of a psychosis. *Prima facie* these confabulations are a psychosis. This is why the syndrome is also sometimes described as Korsakoff's psychosis.

What theories do we have in neuropsychology to explain this syndrome? Obviously, there are controversies and all sorts of diverse opinions. To cut to heart of the matter, most theorists agree that there seem to be two or perhaps three deficits: three parts of the functional architecture of the mind that are, as it were, missing or broken to account for this syndrome. The first is that there must be some disorder of the memory systems. What they specifically say is that these patients have great difficulty in searching their memory stores. Thus there is a deficit of memory search, of finding the correct memory. The second deficit is that the memories that they do actually manage to retrieve with this defective search method, inaccurate though they may be, are not appropriately monitored. This means that there is not an adequate questioning of whether a particular memory is correct or not. The third deficit, which some think is also necessary, is a more general executive abnormality. In other words, they have a more general difficulty in monitoring and organizing their mental processes altogether, in gaining insight and reflecting on the adequacy of their performances. This, very simply stated, is the generic theory that exists in cognitive neuroscience today.

Now what happens when one studies such a patient psychoanalytically, when one takes a patient like this into a psychoanalytic treatment? It must, incidentally, be a psychoanalytic *treatment* that you take such patients into—not only this group of patients but all the patients that we are studying in this way. If one is going to gain access to the inner life of a human being, one needs to try to help the person. One needs to win the person's trust and involvement in the task because without his/her involvement the process is greatly handicapped. Thus, we are trying always to help these patients. Whether we actually do help them is, of course, a moot point. It remains to be seen with future research the extent to which we might be able to help these patients with the really devastating changes in their emotional lives that occur with such lesions. When one gets to know these patients as people, in this way, as opposed to giving them a behavioural checklist or a questionnaire to answer or scoring them against some sort of objective criteria, then something emerges, something that to any psychoanalyst sitting with one of these patients would be absolutely self-evident but which nevertheless is something that is missing from the neuropsychological literature on them. What exactly is missing I shall describe as I proceed. However, what emerges is the fact that these confabulations, random associations, bizarre thoughts, and inventions are, in fact, far from random and far from meaningless. There is an obvious underlying structure and coherence to the train of thoughts that these patients uncontrollably spew out when one listens to them in a psychoanalytic consulting room.

I saw the particular patient with a tumour every day for the past two weeks (six sessions a week). For the first time I tape-recorded the sessions, thinking that it might be useful to capture an objective record. What we were beginning to learn was so interesting, I wanted to be able to demonstrate it. I have, however, been surprised at how disappointing the result of tape-recording is. Reading through the transcript of his extended ramblings, I realized that it really does not convey anything close to what I experienced with the patient. What follows is an excerpt of the transcript of my tenth session with him. I have edited it slightly, cut out some of the "ums" and "aahs" and the stammerings that never went anywhere. This is necessary if it is not to be completely incoherent. It did not feel so incoherent at the time.

Clinical vignette

I had been seeing him for nine days, Monday to Saturday. What I am reporting is the Thursday session of the second week. Each day, he fails to recognize me. He does not know who I am; he has never met me before, as far as he knows. I have nothing to do with brains or minds. I am one thing or another. One day I was a university mate of his, we were in a rowing team together. Another day I was a soccer mate of his; yet another day, a drinking partner. Frequently, I was something to do with his business activity (electronic engineering). I was a client, I was a colleague, I was a business partner, and on this particular Thursday he thinks of me as a doctor. This, I believe, represents progress. The minute that I come down to the consulting room to fetch him, his hand goes up to his head, where he has a scar from the craniotomy, and he says, "Hi Doc!" I was really taken by that. So I go upstairs with him to my consulting room and sit down.

As I sit down I say to him, "You pointed to your head when we met in the consulting room", wanting to try to retain this new development. He says, "I think the problem is a cartridge is missing. We must . . . we just need the specs", by which he means specifications. "We just need the specs. What was it? A C49? Should we order it?" I say, "What does a C49 cartridge do?" He says, "Memory. It's a memory cartridge, a memory implant."

The implant refers to the previous session where I was a dentist in his mind. In reality, he had implants and other dental work done a few years ago. So this immediately comes to my mind. He says, "But I never really understood it. In fact, I haven't used it for a good five or six months now." His surgery, by the way, was about ten months ago. "It seems we don't really need it. It was all chopped away by a doctor, what's his name, a Dr Solms, I think."

Now that is also very interesting because clearly he did not know me from a bar of soap prior to his consulting me after his surgery and after the onset of this amnesia. So there is this name "Dr Solms" somewhere in his head, and it got in there since the onset of his amnesia. "What's his name? Dr Solms I think. But it seems I don't really need it. The implants work fine." So I say to him, "You're aware that something's wrong with your memory but . . ." and he interrupts me and says, "Yes, it's not working one hundred percent, but we don't really need it." Again, I think it is really an enormous step forward for him to recognize that his memory isn't working, let alone knowing that we are talking about memory at all. "Yes, it's not working one hundred percent, but we don't really need it—it was just missing a few beats. The analysis showed that there was some C or C09 missing. Denise brought me here to see a doctor."

Denise, incidentally, is his first wife. He is now remarried and his new wife, who has a different name, is who actually brought him.

He says, "Denise brought me here to see a doctor, what's his name again, Dr Solms or something, and he did one of those heart transplant things and now it's working fine again, never misses a beat." Now he is referring to heart transplants. He did in fact have angioplasty many years before. So he has had some minor heart surgery but obviously not a heart transplant.

I say to him, "You're aware that's something's amiss. Some memories are missing and, of course, that's worrying. You hope I can fix it just like those other doctors fixed the problems with your teeth and your heart. But you want that so much that you're having difficulty accepting that it's not fixed already."

He says, "Oh, I see, yes, it's not working a hundred percent", and he touches his head again. "I got knocked on the head, went off the field for a few minutes but it's fine now. I suppose I shouldn't come back on, but you know me, I don't like going down. So I asked Tim Noakes" (a sports medicine specialist), "so I asked Tim Noakes because I've got the insurance, you know, so why not use it, why not go to the best and he said, fine, play on."

Obviously he is talking about his memory. Although he is talking in fact about all sorts of other things, underneath there is something guiding him, an awareness of his memory loss, which was a new development. I keep trying to point this out to him, that this is what is really worrying him, this is what is really on his mind. Eventually he starts to become a little bit agitated and starts to talk about explosives and says, "Well, in this factory" (now we're in a factory) "there are a lot of detonators lying around and it can be very dangerous and it's, you know, it's not good for youngsters to not follow the correct procedures. There can be an explosion."

I interpret this as his pointing out to me that this is getting dangerous, he is starting to feel very unsettled by what I'm talking about; some emotion is starting to get involved here, it is not just an intellectual matter. I get through to him again, I think, so that again he is focusing. Awareness again dawns on him that he has got a memory disorder and he doesn't know whether he is coming or going. He is really lost. It is extremely distressing. Then he stands up and starts searching in his pockets for a piece of paper which he says he has lost, but there was no piece of paper in his pockets, and I say to him that perhaps he had left it elsewhere; I didn't see him bringing any piece of paper in here. He is searching in his pockets and takes off his trousers and shakes the trouser legs looking for the piece of paper, now in a really agitated state, the sort of state that you get into when you've lost something important, something that really matters to you, and you're looking for it. Then he takes the chair and looks under the chair, picks the chair up, looks under the chair, and I started to feel a little bit concerned, a little bit anxious for my safety with this big guy with a chair in his hands.

I will break off the description of the session there. He was showing me how agitated he was feeling about what he had lost, about the loss of his memory.

Discussion

The experience I have of the patient is that it is like trying to find a radio station or a television channel: you turn the knob and you're just off the station, then you're on the station and it's all in focus and then it goes off again and then there's all this fuzzy sort of noise and then you're just about on the station and you can see the picture flickering and then you know that's the one that you want and you try to tune it back in again, and then you're on it, and then you think thank heavens I'm there, and then it all goes again. That is what his associations are like; that is how it feels to listen to him. He, or at least part of him, is trying to find the real station, the actual memory or the awareness of what is actually happening in his world right now. As he goes onto that station, he cannot stay there, and he goes away again. But he does not go away just anywhere; he goes more or less within that waveband. He is just about on the spot that he is looking for. Thus what he throws up are all these images, thoughts, and memories, which are in some more or less obvious way connected with the thing that he is looking for.

In sum, he is trying to find a certain thing, but what he finds instead is a whole lot of things around it that are *symbolically connected*, one might say, in the broadest sense, to the topic that he is actually looking for. It is like being in a dream, quite literally, as we understand dreams in psychoanalysis, where the images are not random. Underneath or behind these images are other thoughts, which connect them in a coherent way. It is exactly like this with this type of patient, as if they are speaking symbolically or metaphorically, and all one has to do is make these very simple—I almost hesitate to call them—"interpretations", and then you get them back on track again and then they go off again.

That is the first thing one can see by looking at the content of the patient's associations. This is a cognitive account, although we are more interested in the content or meaning than perhaps a cognitive neuroscientist would be. Yet it is more than that. It is not just that the patient's thoughts go off focus. There is clearly something else at work here, which is an emotional factor. This is the second thing we notice. There are certain "wavebands" that he cannot tolerate. He has a reduced tolerance of reality, so that when he becomes aware of the very troubled, disturbing state in which he literally does not know where he is, he cannot retain the focus. This patient does not know what happened a minute ago or who this guy is sitting in front of him, and he cannot bear that awareness of the reality he is in. Another process takes over, a sort of delusional psychotic process, in which he replaces what he observes (if he does manage to observe it) with something that is more bearable and more tolerable to him. Thus, it is not simply a cognitive defect. There is an emotionally based factor too, which accounts for the symptoms that we see in Korsakoff's syndrome. This, I am afraid, is the only discovery (if one can call it that) that we can offer cognitive neuroscience about this syndrome. What one is seeing is not simply a deficit of the machinery of memory. There is something that *rises up* to fill the gap left by that deficit. In short, there is a dynamic interplay. The reality-monitoring part of the mind is weakened, and some other force, which is usually held at bay, rises up, commensurate with the weakening of that reality-monitoring force. This *positive symptomatology* is what I now want briefly to describe.

The type of thinking that rises up in these cases to replace their sense of reality can be summarized under four headings. I shall use some of the patients in the book I mentioned earlier (Kaplan-Solms & Solms, 2000) as examples of these more general points.

1. Replacement of external by psychic reality

First, there is a replacement of external by internal reality. These patients give a disproportionate weight to internal or psychic reality at the expense of material, external, objective reality. An example of this is the patient just described. The objective reality is "brain". That is what we are talking about: brain and memory disorder.

Internally to him, however, these are connected to other images, which have to do with teeth and hearts, and these take precedence over the objective reality. These internal thought processes, connected to the objective topic, are treated as if they too are objectively relevant. I repeat that there is an emotional or wishful factor here too. His teeth and heart were cured. His memory problem is in all likelihood incurable. Thus, in replacing the external reality with an internal one, there is also a shift of a tendentious kind.

Another patient described in our book (Kaplan-Solms & Solms, 2000, Case G, p. 218) was a man who experienced his psychotherapy as if it were a conference. To him, all of these psychotherapy sessions were conference sessions. He saw me (he believed) as part of a course. Moreover, when he was moved from one ward to another in the hospital, he experienced this as being dropped from the football team. This is the memory that it evoked for him: "I'm dropped from a football team." Thus, the internal associations take precedence over the external facts.

Many of these patients described the most amazing things that they did the previous night. These descriptions are an overvaluation of dream experiences, which are then treated as if they too were real experiences.

One patient (Case H, p. 211) was always talking about pyramids and the shifting sands outside the hospital and so on, as if we were in a desert and in Egypt. We subsequently learnt from one of the nurses that he was busy reading a book about the pyramids at Giza. Whereas you and I would read a book and fantasize about being in Egypt, to this man, he was actually in Egypt; his fantasies were just as valid as his actual experience of being in the ward. He also believed that he was in a hotel in the Caribbean while he was in our ward, and that he was on holiday on a barge (Case H, p. 208). Here the theme seems to be confined space, with strangers. Rather than its being a hospital, it is a holiday, the Caribbean, a barge.

2. Exemption from mutual contradiction

Second, there is an excessive tolerance of mutual contradiction. These patients hold two or more things to be true which cannot in fact all be true at the same time. For example, one of the patients

(Case F, p. 203), a woman, believed that the man in the bed next to hers was her husband, and she treated him as her husband. Although he bore no physical resemblance to her husband, she told everyone that he was her husband and she treated him literally like her husband in every way. She also recognized that her husband came and visited her daily, and when her other "husband" was there, they were both her husband and this was quite acceptable to her. She could tolerate the idea of her real husband and this man next door both being her husband at the same time.

One patient had an even more striking tolerance of mutual contradiction (Case H, p. 209). He came excitedly to his therapist, my wife Karen, and said that he had just met in the hospital an old friend of his who died some years ago in Kenya. He was really pleased to have seen him. Once again, in a strange place, the patient recognizes a familiar face. Karen asked him, "But how can you have met him here in the hospital if he died twenty years ago in Kenya?" He stopped for a moment and replied, "Yes, that must present interesting legal problems, being dead in one country and alive in another!" It is notable, and also of theoretical interest, that there is something funny about much of what these patients do. (We have a theory about humour in psychoanalysis, which I think is pertinent in these cases.) Commonly these patients report that relatives of theirs are dead, but at the same time they assert that these relatives are alive. Relatives are simultaneously dead and alive. That is tolerance of mutual contradiction. We even had one patient (Case G, p. 216) who believed that he himself was dead (a contradiction if there ever was one!), telling others about the experience of being dead and still being there to describe it. (One is reminded of the fact that there is no such thing as death in the unconscious.)

3. Timelessness

The third feature of these cases is timelessness. For them, time is not an objective fact but, rather, a theoretical construct that one can use at will. In fact one patient (Case H, p. 209) even said, when contradicted on a certain point about time, "Well, there are many different types of time. There's your time, there's my time, there's adjusted time, there's municipal time, there's hospital time." This is exactly how it is with them. Time can be used in various ways depending on your needs. That same patient always believed it was 5:00 pm, no matter what time of the morning or afternoon or night it was; it was 5:00 pm. If he had just had breakfast, it was 5:00 pm. If he is busy having breakfast, it is 5:00 pm. In fact, 5:00 pm happened to be the time that his wife visited him every day. Thus, the wishful or emotional element is apparent again. As this particular patient was leaving the consulting room, he said to my wife, "Oh, 5:00 pm. You know Buffy's going to be here." I think his wife's name was something like Buffy. Karen replied: "No its not 5:00 pm; its 11:00 am". He then saw a NO SMOKING sign on the wall with a red diagonal line through a circle, which he took to be a clock-face, and said, "Look, *it is* 5:00 pm" pointing to the sign. Once again, wishful inner reality overwhelms external facts.

In fact, achronogenesis—a failure to sequence events in time—is a well-described aspect of this syndrome, even in the cognitive neuroscience literature. What is also seen is a condensation of time. This is not only a failure to order events, but events happening on top of each other, as in the female patient (Case F, p. 203) mentioned before. She had had a hysterectomy, a previous hospital admission, and a deep vein thrombosis in her leg. She described all of these conditions and all three of these hospitals as what was happening to her now: she was here for a hysterectomy, she was here for a brain operation, she was here for a deep vein thrombosis; she was in this hospital, that hospital and the other hospital, all at the same time. Again, one sees the dream-like quality of these patients' thoughts.

4. Primary process (mobility of cathexis)

The last of the four positive features of these cases is a primary-process type of mentation: one object replaces another at will. Depending on the patient's need, a strange man can be your husband if you need him to be your husband; this thing in your head can be a dental procedure if you need it to be a dental procedure. Additionally, there is a visual concretization and objectification of abstract thoughts. The main patient, described initially, was aware that there was something wrong with his memory. He turns it into: "I've lost a piece of paper that was in my pocket which contains specifications." All of the displacements, condensations, visual representations and concretizations evident in these patients are recognizable from dreaming thought. The wishful thread is readily apparent all the way through. I will now take a step backwards and attempt to pull all this together.

Conclusion

What do these observations tell us about the functional architecture of the mind? What is it that this part of the brain does that psychoanalytic study of these patients elucidates and that was not otherwise readily apparent? Alternatively, how can we represent our model, our understanding of the functional architecture of the mind, in this syndrome? What, psychoanalytically speaking, has gone wrong with these patients? I am going to describe in the most rudimentary theoretical terms different psychoanalytic perspectives on this. What I think we see in these patients is the four principal characteristics described above, which are what Freud described as the four "principal characteristics of the system unconscious". His paper on "The Unconscious" (1915e) holds that these four things (1) replacement of external reality by psychical reality, (2) exemption from mutual contradiction, (3) timelessness, and (4) primary process (mobility of cathexis) are the principal functional features of the unconscious. All four characteristics are apparent in these patients. One does not need to infer them: they are there; the unconscious is on the surface, as it were. What theoretical sense can we make of this? It seems that whatever it is that normally suppresses this type of mentation is weakened by a lesion to this part of the brain. Remember: this happens only with damage here. Other brain-damaged patients are different. Something essential to what Freud called the system preconscious or the secondary process, the reality-oriented part of the mind or something essential to it, is missing in these patients. The reality principle breaks down with damage to this part of the brain.

We cannot localize the whole system preconscious in this part of the brain. Yet we know that some function performed by that part of the brain is essential for that entire functional system, which we call the system preconscious, or the secondary process, or the reality principle. With that function removed, what comes through or what replaces it is what Freud called the system unconscious, the primitive, wishful, reality-ignoring aspect of the mind.

This leads to the question posed earlier: what does psychoanalysis add to cognitive neuroscience's description of the cognitive deficits in these cases? We add the realization that their positive symptoms, these more primitive tendencies in the mind that are *released*, account for much of what is actually seen in the symptom complex of Korsakoff's syndrome. It is not simply a matter of *deficit*.

By way of this very simple example, it is possible, using the method of clinico-anatomical correlation, to find a foothold in functional anatomy, in order to link our basic psychoanalytic concepts with the functional anatomy of the brain. I have described just one syndrome and used one theoretical concept to make sense of it. Of course, when one studies all the different syndromes that arise with damage to all different parts of the brain, one gets a much richer picture, a much more fully elaborated theoretical understanding, of what exactly is occurring in each of these syndromes. For example, a release of primary-process types of thinking does not only occur if there are lesions in this area. In different ways, other elements of primary-process thinking occurs with other syndromes. By studying all these syndromes together, we get a picture of what the different aspects are of this broader complex phenomenon that we call secondary-process thought. In the process of doing that, we not only manage to make links between our psychoanalytic theories and physical tissues, with all the scientific advantages that this opens up; we also have the opportunity of understanding in more detail what a global thing like "secondary process" might be in smaller bits. We develop a deeper understanding of what that broad-brushstroke concept is all about. As has happened with all the previous psychological theories that have driven this kind of research, in attempting to correlate our theoretical concepts with functional anatomy, one also finds the flaws and the shortcomings of one's theory. In this way, one can build a better theory of how the mind works. Ultimately, that is the aim of both neuroscientists and psychoanalysts: to build a better theory of how the mind works.

A final point is that what is needed is not simply doing this kind of research but also communicating our findings with neuroscientists, with people on the other side of the divide, working on the same problem. Sadly, in the real world, it is not always the case that they are interested in our work. Historically, neuroscientists have not been interested in psychoanalysis. This kind of research project in which we are involved also entails grappling with how science really works. We have gone to enormous lengths to try to create dialogues between psychoanalysts and neuroscientists, mainly by starting an inter-disciplinary journal, *Neuropsychoanalysis*, with an equal number of leading analysts and neuroscientists on its editorial board. We publish research on topics such as this one, and we hold dialogues in the pages of the journal about our findings and publish psychoanalytic observations on topics of neuroscientific interest. This has been an introduction to a very broad field in which I hope I have managed to interest some of you.

PART III

NEUROPSYCHOANALYTIC PERSPECTIVES ON SOME PSYCHIATRIC DISORDERS

CHAPTER SIX

Depression:
a neuropsychoanalytic perspective

Mark Solms

Introduction

When Sigmund Freud first argued that the mind is not synonymous with consciousness, he was roundly criticized, mainly on philosophical grounds. Subsequent empirical findings have, however, strongly supported his view that many if not most mental functions do not require consciousness to operate effectively (Solms & Turnbull 2002). In fact, the evidence for this view is now so overwhelming that the converse question is being asked: why do we need consciousness at all? This question deeply haunts contemporary efforts to explore and explain the mental functions of the brain.

It is therefore interesting to note that in a posthumously published outline of his life's work, Freud (1940a [1938], p. 157)

This chapter was first published as Solms, M. & Panksepp, J. (2010), "Why depression feels bad", in E. Perry, D. Collerton, F. LeBeau, & H. Ashton (Eds.), *New Horizons in the Neuroscience of Consciousness* (Amsterdam: John Benjamins), pp 169–179; it was republished in a revised version as Solms, M. (2012), "Depression: A neuropsychoanalytic perspective", in *International Forum of Psychoanalysis*, 21: 207–213.

asserted that consciousness was *the most unique characteristic* of the part of nature that we call the mind—"a fact without parallel". The fact of consciousness, Freud wrote, "defies all explanation and description". He continued: "Nevertheless, if anyone speaks of consciousness we know immediately and from our most personal experience what is meant by it". He then added a disparaging remark to the effect that "one extreme line of thought, exemplified in the American doctrine of behaviourism [which was just then coming to prominence], thinks it possible to construct a psychology which disregards this fundamental fact!"

Behaviourism

It is well known why behaviourists wanted to construct a science of the mind that disregarded its most unique characteristic. Consciousness cannot be observed externally; it is not amenable to objective scrutiny. Consciousness is for that reason an embarrassment to science, the ideal of which is objective fact over subjective experience. The behaviourists, who wanted to treat the mind as if it were no different from any other part of nature, therefore ruled consciousness out of court and limited scientific psychology to the study of the objectively observable *outputs* of the mind—to the study of behaviour. Observable experimental manipulations ("stimuli") could then be used to discover the causal mechanisms of behavioural "responses". In this way, the intervening variables (conceptualized as the laws of *learning*) became the only valid objects of psychological science.

Not surprisingly, a school of thought predicated on the assumption that the mind consists in nothing but learning, and disregards all other mental phenomena, centrally including those that we "know immediately and from our most personal experience", was doomed to failure. To deny the causal influence on behaviour of conscious states (like feelings) is to deny the obvious. If one says, that person committed suicide because he could not stand the pain any longer, one is describing the simple causal power of that person's feelings. If one were to try to rephrase this causal statement so as to exclude the feelings, one would be doing violence to the obvious facts.

Thankfully, therefore, in the psychology of the last quarter of a century, realism triumphed over fundamentalism, and consciousness found its way back into science. Even though consciousness still cannot be observed directly, or objectively, today neuroscientists are nevertheless willing to acknowledge its existence in their experimental subjects, and on this basis to infer the causal mechanisms by which conscious states influence behaviours.

Or are they?

The mechanisms of consciousness may be ontologically equivalent to those of learning (or anything else) but the *mechanisms* of consciousness differ in fundamental respects from consciousness *itself*. Mechanisms of all kinds are abstractions, derived from experience; they are not experiences themselves. The mechanisms of consciousness, like all other mechanisms, therefore present no special problems for science; they, too, can be described from an objective standpoint, from the third-person point of view. But this excludes the "fundamental fact" of consciousness—namely, that we *experience* it personally. Is consciousness not perhaps still an embarrassment to science; do neuroscientists today not perhaps still think it possible to construct a psychology that disregards the causal role of this uniquely subjective characteristic of the mind— the fundamental characteristic of this part of nature?

Cognitive neuroscience

It is, in my view, no accident that the apparent re-admittance of consciousness to psychology coincided with advances in the neurosciences which made it possible to study the *physiological correlates* of almost any mental state. By shifting the focus of their research efforts to the physical *correlates* of consciousness, neuroscientists were able to pay lip service to its existence without having to trouble themselves too much with its intrinsically subjective nature— with the original source of the embarrassment. Small wonder, then, that so many behaviourists made such a seamless transition to the new paradigm.

As Freud put it:

> there would thus be no alternative left to assuming that there are physical or somatic processes which are concomitant with the psychical ones and which we should necessarily have to recognize as more complete than the psychical sequences. . . . [Then] it of course becomes plausible to lay the stress in psychology on those somatic processes, to see in *them* the true essence of what is psychical. [1940a (1938), p. 157)

To seek the essence of what is "psychical" in something that lacks its most unique property is surely to look in the wrong place. But this does not mean that we must abandon reality. Nor does it mean (today) that the brain is the wrong place to seek an understanding of consciousness. It means only that we must admit that consciousness actually exists, that it is a property of nature, that it is a property of the part of nature called the brain or mind (depending on your observational perspective; see Solms, 1997a), and that this property is no less real and no less causally efficacious than any other natural properties. This in turn means that we must recognize that the brain is not *quite* the same as every other part of nature. The brain has some special properties, and central among these is consciousness. As a consequence of it being conscious, the brain behaves differently from most other things, even from other bodily organs.

As far as I can tell, despite appearances, these views are still not generally accepted, or at least they are not generally incorporated in the current theoretical paradigms of cognitive neuroscience. In fact the very power of cognitive neuroscience seems to be that it treats the organ of the mind as if it were no different from any other bodily organ, indeed from any other complex mechanism—living or dead.

Biological psychiatry

The baneful consequences of this continued neglect of the "fundamental fact" of consciousness have been more evident in the field of biological psychiatry than in cognitive neuroscience in general. This is perhaps not surprising, because psychiatry is all about feelings. (How else does it differ from neurology?)

In psychiatry today, if one says: the patient committed suicide because he could not stand the pain any longer, one seems to mean: the patient *thought* he was committing suicide because he could not stand the pain any longer, but *really* he was committing suicide because his serotonin levels were depleted (or something like that). The point is: what the patient says, thinks, or feels may be left out of our scientific account; the feelings evidently are not really part of the causal chain of events. They are just a layperson's translation of the actual state of affairs in the brain. This, in my view, is doing violence to the facts. In my view, the feelings are a fundamental part of the actual state of affairs.

I shall now illustrate these principles with reference to a particular problem in modern psychiatry, namely: what is depression for? By this I mean: what is the *feeling* complex that is the core feature of depression for; why does this unique quality of conscious that we called "depressed" exist; what does it do?

In fact, this problem is not even posed in psychiatry. It is not posed because what depression feels like does not matter in contemporary psychiatric science, even though it is officially classified as a *mood* disorder. This is evidently because feelings in general do not matter. What matters is the physical *correlates* of the feelings: the brain states and other physiological variables that *accompany* depression. This approach, in my view, is based on a serious misconception of how the brain works, which will almost inevitably lead to big mistakes.

In their haste to avoid the embarrassingly subjective phenomena of depression, psychiatric researchers have in recent decades focused on all sorts of things that correlate with depression, or facilitate it, or contextualize it—and the neural mechanisms of those things—rather than the nature of depression itself.

The main focus of depression research for the past three decades has been the neurophysiological mechanisms of *serotonin depletion* (Harro & Oreland, 2001; Schildkraut, 1965), including the neurotrophic effects of this depletion (Koziek, Middlemas, & Bylund, 2008), the neuroendocrinological mechanisms of stress (which have similar neurotrophic consequences; De Kloet, Joels, & Holsboer,

2005), the neuroimmunological equivalents of these mechanisms (McEwen, 2007), their interactions with sleep mechanisms (Zupancic & Guilleminault, 2006), their genetic underpinnings (Levinson, 2006), and so on.

These research programmes have evidently been followed because the mechanisms of serotonin depletion (and its cognates) are eminently tractable scientific problems—notwithstanding the fact that they have nothing to do with actually researching depressive feelings. The reason these programmes have been followed cannot possibly be because the researchers concerned seriously think that depressive feelings (let alone major depression) are actually *caused* by low levels of serotonin. There is very little evidence for that. In fact, it is well established that experimental depletion of brain serotonin does not cause depression (Delgado et al., 1990). Nor was there ever any reason to believe that serotonin *would* play any such specific causal role in depressive mood. Serotonin is an all-purpose modulator of moods and emotions, not only of depressive ones (Berger, Gray, & Roth, 2009). It is probably for this reason that SSRIs (selective serotonin reuptake inhibitors) are used to treat not only depression but also a host of other emotional troubles, such as panic attacks and obsessive compulsive disorder. This is also probably the reason why SSRIs do *not* work in so many cases of depression, and why they work only partially or temporarily in the vast majority of cases (cf. STAR*D [sequenced treatment alternatives to relieve depression] findings). The same applies to the various physiological cascades associated with serotonin depletion: stress or inflammation or hippocampal shrinkage. None of these things has a specific causal relationship with depression. They are too general; "too much" of an explanation. Their main attraction is only that they are scientifically tractable and therefore scientifically respectable mechanisms.

In summary, it is clear that although the mechanisms of serotonin depletion and its cognates correlate with or facilitate or contextualize depression, something else—something far more specific—must be the actual causal mechanism of depression. I suggest that this "something else" most likely has something to do with the brain mechanisms that actually generate depressive *feelings*.

Depression itself

My reason for suggesting this is the fact that the clinical phenomenology of depression is characterized above all else by a complex
of feelings: low mood, low self-esteem, loss of motivation and
energy, sense of guilt, loss of pleasure in the world, and so on. Is
this feeling complex not the most obvious place to seek the essential
nature of depression? And dare we ask whether this constellation
of feelings *means* anything? It is after all in the essential nature of
feelings that they mean something. It would be entirely normal
and reasonable for all of us (even for scientists) to ask—outside
our clinical or scientific work—what it might mean when people
say that they feel down, bad, defeated, useless; that they have lost
all hope for themselves, lost all interest in other people, and so on.
Why do they feel this?, we would normally ask. Certainly it is *possible* that these feelings are meaningless epiphenomena of a brain
disease called "depression"—even though they give the disease its
name and even though feelings are not normally meaningless—but
it is at least equally possible (and in my view more so) that they
are *not* meaningless.

I think the most obvious way of making meaningful sense of this
complex of feelings is suggested by what the *DSM-IV* (APA, 1994)
definition of major depression describes as diagnostic criterion E:

> The symptoms are not better accounted for by bereavement. [empha-
> sis added]

This differential diagnostic criterion suggests that depression may
be easily mistaken for bereavement, which in turn suggests that
depression is characterized by a complex of feelings that closely
resembles those associated with grief. Normally, this complex of
feelings tends to mean: "I am bereaved." It therefore seems reasonable to infer that the disorder called depression might have
something to do with *loss*. This reminds us of what the early psychological investigators of depression (who were not embarrassed
by feelings and their meanings) concluded on the basis of *talking*
to patients about what their feelings might mean: they concluded
that depression was akin to grief, that it seemed in fact to be a
pathological form of *mourning* (Freud, 1917e [1915]).

It is in fact well established today that early separation experiences do indeed predispose to depression (Heim & Nemeroff, 1999; Pryce et al., 2005), possibly through mediation of the stress cascades that McEwen (2000) has identified, and possibly also via other "general sickness" mechanisms (McEwen, 2007). We also know that a first depressive episode is most likely to be triggered by social loss (Bowlby, 1980), and so on. In other words, both the psychoanalytic evidence and the ethological evidence point to the same common-sense observation—namely, that depressed feelings have something to do with attachment and loss.

Affective neuroscience

In light of such commonplace observations to the effect that depressive feelings are connected with the psychology of attachment and loss, why are cognitive neuroscientists *not* focusing their attention on the mammalian brain systems that evolved specifically for the purpose of mediating attachment and loss, and which produce the particular type of pain associated with these biological phenomena of universal significance—namely, *separation distress* (also known as "protest" or "panic"), which, if it does not result in reunion, is typically followed by hopeless "despair".

It is well-established that a specific mammalian brain system evolved precisely to generate these depression-like feelings (Panksepp, 1998a, 2003b, 2005b). This brain system evolved from general pain mechanisms more than 200 million years ago, apparently for the purpose of forging long-term *attachments* between mothers and their offspring, between sexual mates, and ultimately between social groups in general. When such social bonds are broken through separation or loss of a loved one, or the like, then these brain mechanisms make the sufferer feel bad in a particular way. This special type of pain is called separation distress or panic. The biological value of this type of pain is that it motivates the sufferer to avoid separation, and to *seek reunion* with the lost object. However, if this biologically desirable outcome fails to materialize, then a second mechanism kicks in, which shuts down the distress and causes the lost individual to *give up*. This giving up is the "despair" phase of

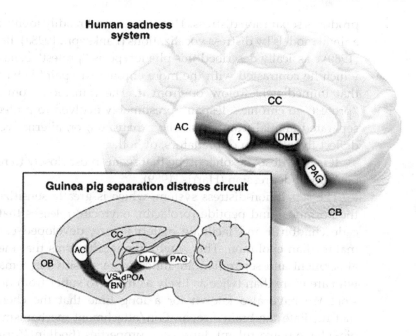

FIGURE 6. 1.   The separation-distress system. AC = anterior cingulate gyrus; BN = bed nucleus of the stria terminalis; CB = cerebellum; CC = corpus callosum; DMT = dorsomedial thalamus; dPOA = dorsal preoptic area; OB = olfactory bulb; PA = periaqueductal grey; VS = ventral striatum. (From Panksepp, 2003b.)

social loss (Panksepp, Lensing, & Bernatzky, 1989; Panksepp, Yates, Ikemoto, & Nelson, 1991).

This system is embodied in a well-defined network of brain structures (Figure 6.1), starting in the anterior cingulate gyrus (about which so much has been said in recent neuro-imaging studies and deep brain stimulation treatments of depression; Mayberg et al., 2005), coursing downwards through various thalamic, hypothalamic, and other basal forebrain nuclei, terminating in the ancient midbrain (pain-generating) neurons of the PAG. Activation and deactivation of this system is fundamentally mediated by opioid receptors. Mu-opioid agonists in particular activate it in such a way as to generate feelings of secure well-being that are the very opposite of depression, whereas mu-opioid blockade or withdrawal produces separation distress. This state is most readily identified in animal models by distress vocalizations (Panksepp, 1998a). Bowlby (1980) classically described this phenotype as "protest" behaviour, which he contrasted with the more chronic "despair" behaviours that immediately follow on from it. The transition from acute "protest" to chronic "despair" presumably evolved to protect the separated animal from metabolic exhaustion, or, alternatively, to deflect the attention of predators, or both.

It is the "despair" phenotype that seems most closely to resemble clinical depression (Harris, 1989).

The separation-distress system, which is greatly sensitized by the hormonal and peptide (prolactin, oxytocin) releases that precede childbirth and facilitate maternal care, developed early in mammalian evolution. This is why the mechanisms that mediate attachment and separation are much more sensitive in females— who are more than twice as likely as males to suffer from depression. We have also known for a long time that the chemicals that mediate the brain's separation/attachment mechanism (opioids) have powerful antidepressant properties (Bodkin, Zornberg, Lukas, & Cole, 1995). If it were not for the addictive risks of opiates, they would almost certainly have formed the front line of antidepression medications. In fact, there is good reason to believe that the natural brain chemicals—endorphins—that make us feel good when we are safely and securely attached are themselves addictive; in short, that affectionate bonds are a primal form of addiction. This system apparently provides the elemental means by which mother and infant attach to each other—the means by which they become addicted to one another.

Although these opioid-driven attachment systems may be the pivotal mechanism that produces depression, there are many intermediate mechanisms that generate the various depressive subtypes. Central to these is dynorphin-facilitated shutdown of dopamine-driven appetitive systems, which is when the individual "gives up" in despair (Nestler & Carlezon, 2006).

It seems that the pain of social loss and defeat are the price that we mammals had to pay for the evolutionary advantages bestowed by this opioid-mediated system—that is, by mammalian social attachment, the prototype of which is the mother–infant bond. This is an instance of a more general principle: conscious feelings, both positive and negative, evolved because *they enhance survival and reproductive success*. This is their causal role. This is why feelings matter.

Psychoanalysis

The evolutionary processes that gave rise to such emotional endophenotypes as the attachment/loss system do not coincide with the experiences that they produce in the individual. The basic subcortical mechanisms in question should also not be confused with their higher cortical representations and elaborations.

An infant in the grip of separation distress does not think "this loss of my beloved mother is bad for me because it endangers my survival and thereby reduces my reproductive fitness". What the individual feels and thinks may *ultimately* subserve these interests of the species, but what the individual itself experiences is its own self-interest, not the biological mechanisms that gave rise to it. The infant simply feels *bad*; so it cries, trying to get rid of the feeling. Later, to the extent that it develops reflexive cognition, it will come to think things like: "This loss of my beloved mother is bad for me; I therefore want her back." But this subjective experience is still ignorant of the underlying, objective mechanism.

Individuals are motivated primarily by feelings, and secondarily by thoughts, not by mechanisms. This is true even though the objective mechanisms explain (and cause) the subjective feelings and thoughts. People live their lives; they do not live evolutionary biology.

Here is a more complex example: the objective mechanism of the "despair" phase of the separation response appears to be a shutdown of the "protest" (or PANIC) phase, with its associated SEEKING impulses.[1] From the biological standpoint, this prevents metabolic exhaustion, the risk of attracting predatory interest, and the dangers of straying too far from home base. From the neurochemical point of view, this shutdown is mediated by dynorphin blockade of dopamine arousal, which (in behaviourist terms) replaces positive approach behaviours with negative withdrawal behaviours. In learning-theory terms, the seeking of "rewards" thus elicits "punishment" responses.

Psychoanalytic investigations reveal that depression also entails feelings of rage, apparently inwardly-directed but originally directed toward external objects. From the affective-neuroscience standpoint, this is probably due to frustrations of SEEKING desires, which normally elicit RAGE responses (Panksepp, 1998a). The RAGE response in depression, however, seems to be inhibited, or even internalized. This is presumably part of the self-"punishment" mechanism described above. The important thing is that the existence of (inhibited or internalized) RAGE responses in depression would not have been recognized without psychoanalytic investigations.

Nevertheless, subjectively, the whole complicated mechanism results in the simple fact that hopeful feelings are replaced by feelings of hopelessness. Or worse: hope is replaced by an attack on the self, by a punishment of hopefulness, leading to the so-called "negative therapeutic reaction".

The fact that such processes might, at the representational level, involve a denial of the loss of the object, and might thus be pictured as an attack upon an internalized frustrating object, is neither here nor there from the viewpoint of affective neuroscience. The objective mechanism that explains (and ultimately causes) this state of affairs is the survival advantage of a shift from "protest" to "despair", in which the conscious *feelings* play the pivotal role. The representational elaboration of this shift—the internalized attack, producing self-hatred—is almost certainly derived from the underlying instinctual mechanism. (Our human representational capacity for "confabulation" is seemingly endless!) But reflexive cognition is also the route by which an individual comes to know what is happening inside him/herself. It is the only way we can know ourselves, however indirectly. It should therefore not be despised.

For if the example of depression has taught us anything it is this: depression is first and last an internal state, a feeling complex, something *subjective*. This is the most essential ontological feature of depression. This is what makes it real. This is what gives it effect.

The rest is detail.

Conclusion

So what is depression for? And why does it feel bad? It serves a purpose and feels bad, on my hypothesis, for two reasons: first, to encourage us to form attachments, particularly to early care-giving figures, but also with our sexual mates and offspring and social groups and the like; and, second, to persuade us to give up hope if our attempts to reunite with such figures or groups do not succeed within a limited time-frame, when we have become detached (or lost). The fact that such feelings can be too easily provoked, or too difficult to erase, and so on, in some individuals, is immaterial to the biological forces that selected them into the mammalian genome in the first place. The fact that some people have more or less sensitive hearing tells us nothing about the evolution of the auditory sense.

In light of the existence of brain structures that generate depressive feelings, it seems reasonable to at least hypothesize that the linchpin of depression is none of the things that have so preoccupied contemporary psychiatric researchers over the past three decades, but, rather, the evolutionarily conserved brain state that mediates the transition from "protest" to "despair" in the wake of social loss. In other words, it seems reasonable to hypothesize that the core brain basis of depression revolves around the process by which separation distress is normally shut down (by kappa-opioids like dynorphin), prompting the animal to "give up".

Why aren't psychiatric researchers investigating the role of these brain processes in depression? Such processes seem to be the obvious place to start if we are going to take the phenomenology of depression itself (as opposed to things that correlate with it) as our starting point.

We believe that such obvious starting points are neglected due to an ongoing, deep prejudice against acknowledging the implica- •
tions for science of the subjective nature of consciousness, and its causal efficacy in the brain. This coincides with a neglect of the *meaning* of mental states in general. This prejudice is most unfortunate, because subjective consciousness certainly exists, and it almost certainly evolved for a reason (it almost certainly enhances reproductive fitness). It is accordingly almost certainly a central

feature of how the brain works. We therefore ignore it at our peril.

Psychoanalysis—the science of subjective experience—has much to offer neuroscience.

Note

1. The use of capital letters here follows Panksepp's (1998a) usage, to indicate that PANIC and SEEKING, etc., are instinctual emotion systems. Seven such systems have been identified in the mammalian brain. The difference between "panic" and "PANIC," etc., in the terminology of affective neuroscience is analogous to the difference in psychoanalytic terminology between "me" and "the ego".

CHAPTER SEVEN

Neuropsychoanalytic notes on addiction

Mark Solms, Eleni Pantelis, & Jaak Panksepp

F reud had remarkably little to say about addiction, save for this one observation, made early in his psychological work (and often repeated thereafter):

> It has dawned on me that masturbation is the one major habit, the "primal addiction" and that it is only as a substitute and replacement for it that the other addictions—for alcohol, morphine, tobacco, etc.,—come into existence. [Freud, 1950 (1892–1899), p. 272]

A minor elaboration of this view is the following one, also made early in Freud's work:

> Not everyone who has occasion to take morphia, cocaine, chloral-hydrate, and so on, for a period, acquires in this way an "addiction" to them. Closer enquiry usually shows that these narcotics are meant to serve—directly or indirectly—as a substitute for a lack of sexual satisfaction. [Freud, 1898a, p. 276]

This chapter was first published as Solms, M., Pantelis, E., & Panksepp, J. (2012), "Neuropsychoanalytic notes on addiction", in G. Ellis, D. Stein, E. Meintjies, & K. Thomas (Eds.), *Substance Use and Abuse in South Africa* (Cape Town: University of Cape Town Press), pp. 175–184.

In other words, during development masturbation is normally replaced by adult sexual satisfaction, but where it is not it may be substituted by (another) addiction.

These are quintessentially Freudian claims, museum-quality examples of the type. For that reason, perhaps, they are all too easily dismissed by addiction researchers today. If readers are willing to suspend judgement for a moment though, and permit us to unpack the meaning of these claims and reconsider them in the light of contemporary neuroscience, their patience will be amply repaid.

For all of his failings, Freud had an uncanny ability to identify the essence of a psychological problem. The fundamental problem of addiction exposed by the parallel that Freud drew with masturbation is that substance abuse (like masturbation) is an affectively rewarding activity that serves no biological purpose. Substance abuse generates hedonically positive affects in the brain (or reduces negative ones) but does not sustain reproductive fitness. In fact, it does the opposite. Addiction therefore cannot be an evolutionarily proper use of the brain mechanisms in question, but it is psychologically compelling nonetheless.

Substance abuse appears to employ brain mechanisms that were evolutionary designed to reward biologically useful activities (like copulation, as opposed to masturbation). This is what pleasurable affects are *for*, evolutionarily speaking: they reward biologically useful actions, and thus motivate animals to perform the work that is necessary to achieve them (Damasio, 1999b; Solms & Nersessian, 1999). The word "abuse" in substance abuse refers to the fact that the pleasure is attained without the natural effort and persistence it was designed to reward. The motivation to perform the effortful work to achieve biologically useful goals in an indifferent and even hostile world is substituted by mere self-administration of pleasure-producing (or unpleasure-reducing) substances. This requires hardly any effort at all, aside from acquiring drugs that are not legally available, and nothing biologically useful is achieved by it. The prize is thus attained without actually taking part in the competition. The biological purpose of reward is cheated.

Herein presumably lies the root of our moral condemnation of both masturbation and addiction alike.

This conclusion seems to be the implication of the second Freud quotation above: substance abuse (like masturbation) is a biologically/morally inferior *substitute* for "real" sources of satisfaction (like copulation). Substance abuse, like masturbation, represents a failure to negotiate the transition from self-soothing to mastery of the real external world—the arena of all the competitions that we simply have to enter in order to survive and reproduce. Substance abuse, like masturbation, is a biological dead-end.

This begs the question: why and how do we normally negotiate this transition? What enables us to give up effortless masturbatory/addictive pleasures in favour of real ones, in favour of the biologically (and morally) wholesome ones? If we can trace the mechanism by which we normally traverse this transition, we will have identified the pivotal locus of the biological failure (of the psychopathology) called addiction.

It seems unlikely that evolution would have left this important task to moral persuasion (education or learning) alone. There must be some intrinsic mechanism that motivates us to forego empty pleasures in favour of the more difficult and risky business of engagement with the real world. And there does appear to be just such an intrinsic mechanism, the identification of which reveals important shortcomings in many contemporary conceptualizations of the neural basis of reward.

If the biology of reward entailed a unitary brain mechanism, such as the one that many eminent researchers still seem to claim for the mesocortical-mesolimbic dopamine (DA) "reward system" (Haber & Knutson, 2009; Rolls, 1999), then it is difficult to imagine why animals would ever bother to negotiate the task just mentioned. Why not just go straight for the reward and by-pass the effort and risk involved in the activities that "properly" generate them? It comes as no surprise to us to learn, therefore, that the mammalian brain does contain a more complex reward mechanism, which drives us to seek our pleasures in the external world. This latter mechanism is indeed the mesocortical-mesolimbic DA system, but it turns out not to be a simple "reward" system at all—despite the fact that *almost all drugs of abuse* (like all forms of appetitive behaviour) *do indeed massively increase DA activity in this system.*

The mistaken attribution of simple reward functions to the mesolimbic-mesocortical DA system was first appreciated by Panksepp (1982, 1986). He observed that artificial stimulation of this (D2-receptor-mediated) motivational DA system does not generate pleasurable feelings and blissful satiation in mammals—as *consummation* of a need normally should. Rather, it impels the animal to excitedly *seek more of the stimulation* (in other words, it actually increases the *appetitive* drive that *leads* us to rewards, rather than the consummation behaviour that actually *delivers* them). This and subsequent research led Panksepp to rename the DA "reward" system as a "SEEKING" system (Panksepp, 1998a; capitals in the original). The SEEKING system motivates animals to engage with the world—to eagerly forage, to curiously explore, to optimistically expect; in short, to look to the outside world for attaining pleasurable experiences. The SEEKING system is stimulated into action by medial hypothalamic "need-detector" mechanisms, and when it is activated it impels the animal to engage with the real objects that satisfy its inner needs, which *in turn* generate pleasurable experiences via the PLEASURE–LUST system (and other systems), which utilize the SEEKING system for their hedonic ends but which are not themselves primarily mediated by DA. These systems are discussed below.

Berridge and Robinson (1998) were driven to very similar conclusions by their own research findings, which eventually led Berridge (2007) to draw an analogous (but as we shall see, not identical) distinction between the brain mechanisms for "wanting" and "liking" in mammals, with "wanting" being just one step removed from SEEKING. (A full history of the diversity of views in this theoretical hornet's nest is summarized in Alcaro, Huber, and Panksepp, 2007, and in Panksepp & Moskal, 2008.)

It is not difficult to see, in light of our reflections on Freud's observations, why an instinctual SEEKING or "wanting" mechanism would have evolved alongside the PLEASURE or "liking" mechanism. It is a sad but incontrovertible fact that all our needs cannot be met narcissistically, by mere *feelings* of reward versus *actual achievement* of reward. Biological needs represent a true *lack* in the organism that can only be rectified by an object (and usually a rather specific object) in the outside world. This is one of the great facts of life, and an ultimate source of all our struggles.

The distinction between the brain's appetitive and consummatory "reward" mechanisms helps to make sense of the fact that addicts do not generally find their substance-induced DA surges to be pleasurable; at times they do not even *like* the objects of their addictive *wants* (Kassel, 2010).

Most recent addiction research into the "wanting" aspect of the brain's so-called reward mechanisms has, however, not been interpreted within Panksepp's framework as summarized above. It has been interpreted on the view that "wanting" is equivalent to something quite different from simple SEEKING, something called "incentive salience" (Robinson & Berridge, 2003). On this view, DA activity is said to *predict* which objects are likely to produce pleasurable experiences (incentive), and thereby to motivate the animal to selectively attend to such objects (salience). Addiction researchers who follow this view (e.g., Baler & Volkow, 2009) accordingly argue that drug-induced DA surges make addicts over-incentivize the drugs that generate such surges—to consider them excessively important (inappropriately salient).

A moment's thought, however, reveals a significant conflation in this view. Drug-induced surges in salience attribution should incentivize the addicts to pay extra attention to the *pleasure-generating* things they come across while high, not to the thing (the DA agonist) that merely induced the high. On Berridge's own theory, the DA agonist is not intrinsically pleasure generating. The incentive salience theory therefore erroneously treats the DA agonist as if it were itself the reward (the "liking"), which it is not. The foraging behaviours (and the associated curious, interested, expectant, optimistic feelings) that DA actually induce merely increase the chances of the animal encountering the real objects of their needs—the objects that they "like". This, a second stage that can only follow the primary "SEEKING/wanting" process, is what is actually rewarding.

The incentive salience mechanism that Berridge and others attribute to the mesolimbic-mesocortical DA system must therefore be a *third* stage in a complex process. First, the animal has to (1) be driven to seek the objects of its biological needs in the outside world, surely an invigorating hedonic activity, before it can (2) experience the pleasurable rewards that such objects generate, which in turn enables the animal to (3) learn from such experiences—that is, associate specific objects with the pleasurable relief of each need. Only then can the animal have any basis for predicting biologically appropriate pleasures from the sight or smell of specific objects (i.e., attribute incentive salience).

Panksepp, by contrast, has always emphasized the intrinsically "objectless" quality of the SEEKING instinct, calling it "a goad without a goal" (Panksepp, 1971). Learning comes later and involves much more than instinct; learning is a by-product of the encounter between instinct and environment. Learning would therefore never occur if it were not for the existence of a primary instinct towards engagement with the environment—with all the effort, frustration, and risk that this entails.

"Incentive salience"—the learning mechanism—therefore reveals itself to be (in Freudian terms) an "ego" rather than an "id" mechanism. Ironically, this is also where moral persuasion (the "superego") may enter the equation. It is no accident that recent research on the role of incentive salience in addiction has strongly emphasized the contribution in addictive pathogenesis of aberrant *inhibitory controls* on the underlying mesolimbic-mescortical DA activity (Baler & Volkow, 2006). All the influences exerted by parents, upbringing, education, and the like have their effects on these higher ("learning") aspects of the transition from self-soothing to object mastery. We should therefore be on our guard against overly reductionist attempts to elucidate the basic molecular mechanisms of incentive salience conditioning (Chen, Chen, & Chiang, 2009) as being the same as the primary-process motivation employed in SEEKING resources. The variability contributed to any psychopathology by higher order environmental factors such as parenting, upbringing, and education, as Freud taught us, can be very complicated indeed.

It is to the first two steps in the three-step process outlined above that we must return, then, if we wish to elucidate the hard-wired, instinctual ("id") mechanisms leading from self-soothing to object mastery. There are very special hedonic feeling components to the instinctual systems that support those aspects of survival that require a confrontation with the real world.

We have said already that the first step in the process must be a basic SEEKING tendency, which drives the animal to "forage" in the outside world, triggered by its detection of an inner need. Why, then, is this simple and primary DA-activated process so heavily implicated in addiction? After all, SEEKING is the step in the putative process that leads the animal *away* from self-soothing (from Freud's "masturbation"); why then do substances of abuse *increase* activation of this DA mechanism? Does this not reveal a contradiction in the parallel that Freud drew between masturbation and addiction (which he saw as a fixation upon or regression to self-soothing)?

It certainly would be a contradiction if it were not for the important finding (made in relation to cocaine addiction in the 1980s, and in subsequent studies in relation to methamphetamine, alcohol, and heroin, too) that D2 receptors are consistently *decreased* in addicts, even long after the resolution of acute withdrawal effects (Volkow, Fowler, Wang, & Swanson, 2004; Volkow et al., 1990, 1993). Recent research has also shown that relatively decreased D2 receptors *precede* the development of an addiction—that it may in fact be an important biological marker of addictive vulnerability (Nader et al., 2006; Volkow, Fowler, Wang, Swanson, & Telang, 2007; Volkow et al., 2006).

These findings are currently being interpreted to mean that individuals with blunted capacity to attribute "incentive salience" gradually come to learn that only substances that can produce massive surges of D2-mediated activity are salient. But in light of what has been said above against the salience attribution theory, a better interpretation might be that individuals with blunted SEEKING capacities come to learn (especially if not otherwise helped by parents, educators, and the like) that substances that produce massive surges of D2-mediated activity enable them to *gain access to pleasurable experiences and objects in the outside world* that would otherwise be relatively inaccessible to them. The object of the addiction would then be not just the stimulant substance itself—as incentive salience theory suggests—but, rather, the possibility (or expectation, or even hope) of social, sexual, and other biologically useful rewards that the substance artificially evokes. This alternative explanation of the link between reduced D2 receptivity and addiction has important clinical implications, so we believe it deserves careful consideration in future research.

For now, however, coming full circle, it appears that the main focus of the addiction process must still fall back on *pleasurable reward itself.* This, and not the primary SEEKING instinct or the drugs that stimulate it (or the paraphernalia associated with those drugs), seems to remain the ultimate object of addiction. Pleasure (or its habituation, and hence relief from the pain) is still the big-ticket item, as we have seen, the final common pathway.

We have also said already that the PLEASURE–LUST or "liking" aspect of the reward process is not just DA mediated (although DA has a role to play in it). It is generally accepted on current knowledge that the main aspect of the PLEASURE process is mediated by opioids (acting on mu- and delta-receptors in the basal fore-brain region in particular; see Berridge, 1996; Panksepp, 1998a). These are very ancient brain molecules, which are thought to have evolved in the brain initially for their *hedonic* properties, but they also served endogenous *analgesic* functions and therefore came later to ameliorate the behaviourally more complex *pain of social loss* (Panksepp, 1998a). This latter instinctual mechanism—which Panksepp calls the PANIC–GRIEF system—is especially highly developed in mammals, which are exquisitely social animals (but the mechanism must have evolved earlier as it is also present in birds). This system has its epicentre in a neuronal network that courses between anterior cingulate gyrus and various diencephalic nuclei and the dorsal PAG.

The hedonic, analgesic, and social-soothing properties of opioids are difficult to separate entirely, especially when considered from the lived viewpoint of what a substance abuser is trying to achieve. A diagnostic differentiation of this kind would certainly be clinically important, as indeed is the more basic distinction we have already drawn between those who are seeking DA stimulation and those who are seeking opioid-mediated euphoria or relief (cf. "uppers" versus "downers"). But now we must finally consider the opioid systems as a whole in relation to the Freudian formulation of addiction that we are considering here.

It is easy to see the link between an opiate-induced hedonic fog and the narcissistic delights of masturbation. We have likewise already provided an answer to the question as to why animals take the trouble to transcend masturbation and engage instead with the outside world in pursuit of pleasure and relief from pain. The answer was found in the fact that a primary SEEKING instinct exists, alongside various PLEASURE–LUST instincts. This implies that masturbatory pleasure, while satisfying the second of these instincts, leaves the first of them (the object-seeking one) unsatisfied. All at once, this insight throws the pivotal role of the other opioid-mediated instinct, the PANIC–GRIEF one, into sharp relief.

As already mentioned, this system evolved in order to foster social bonds—first and foremost between infants and their mothers, then between sexual mates, and ultimately between social groups of all kinds (including families and clans). It is easy to see the adaptive advantages of such an instinct, which attaches mothers (and to a lesser extent, fathers) to their genetic offspring, the offspring to their major sources of survival care, and genetically related conspecifics more broadly to each other. The price we have to pay for this evolutionary advantage, though, is the pain of social loss: separation distress (PANIC), sadness, and despair (GRIEF). The avoidance of such pain is what keeps us together: neurochemically speaking, we cling to our mothers and lovers in order to keep our mu-opioid receptor activity contentedly high.

Now, it is of the utmost importance to note that the "attachment" processes initiated by this instinctual system *have all the hallmarks of addiction*. Consider for a moment the tabulation of the similarities between social attachment/loss and substance addiction/withdrawal in Table 7.1. The analogies are extremely striking.

Table 7.1.   Similarities between opiate addiction and social dependence

Opiate addiction	Social dependence
1) Drug dependence	1) Social bonding
2) Drug tolerance	2) Estrangement
3) Drug withdrawal	3) Separation distress
a) PSYCHIC PAIN ──────────▶	a) LONELINESS
b) LACRIMATION ──────────▶	b) CRYING
c) ANOREXIA ──────────▶	c) LOSS OF APPETITE
d) DESPONDENCY ──────────▶	d) DEPRESSION
e) INSOMNIA ──────────▶	e) SLEEPLESSNESS
f) AGGRESSIVENESS ──────────▶	f) IRRITABILITY

It comes as no surprise to learn, therefore, that opiates were histori-
cally the first line of treatment for depression (for summary, see
Tenore, 2008). Why, then, did we stop using them for this purpose?
For the simple reason that they are so addictive!

So, *attachment is a primary form of addiction*. Anyone who has
fallen in love knows the truth of this statement. Being in love with
someone is almost indistinguishable from being addicted to them.
This, surely, then, is the biological endophenotype that is high-
jacked by substance abuse.

But where does this leave Freud's claim regarding masturbation? In our view it encourages us to take a deeper view of what
masturbation actually entails. Although it is difficult to know what
is going on in the mind of a masturbating infant (it is important
to remember that Freud included pre-genital pleasures—thumb-
sucking, etc.—under this heading), it seems unlikely that it entails
pleasurable sensations alone, devoid of representational contents.
Certainly this applies to the masturbatory fantasies of adolescents
and adults; what excites the pleasurable sensations is not manual
stimulation alone but almost invariably the presence of an imaginary partner, or at least of another person of some kind. In short,
what distinguishes masturbation from actual copulation is not so
much an absence of object-seeking as a *frustration* of object-seeking.
One masturbates for *lack* of an object (whatever the reason for that
lack might be). This is why masturbation is considered inferior
to copulation, not only by society, but by the masturbator too.
Masturbation is ultimately an empty source of pleasure, in a very
literal sense. Masturbation involves frustration of the SEEKING
instinct, plus satisfaction of the PLEASURE–LUST instinct, which
equals empty (objectless) pleasure; pleasure without attachment, or
worse: substitutive pleasure in the absence of a specific longed-for
object (i.e., subject of affection). This formulation fits perfectly with
the understanding of addiction outlined above. Addiction, like
masturbation, is a substitute and replacement not only for general
mastery of the object world, but specifically for the attainment of
a secure love-object.

This blindingly obvious insight has massive clinical relevance,
today as much as ever. Moreover, the distinction between the abuse
of DA-activating substances to buttress object-seeking, and the

abuse of opiates to actually replace the object, suggests that the latter may be a more malignant (less hopeful) form of addiction.

Despite all Freud's quaint and sometimes misleadingly idiosyncratic language, we trust that readers will agree that his conception of addiction as a substitute for mature sexual love, and therefore an equivalent of masturbation, still describes the pivot of the problem. The deeper and more detailed insights (and potentially powerful new therapeutic tools) provided by modern neuroscientific approaches to the underlying mechanisms around which the problem of addiction revolves, make it all the more imperative that we do not lose sight of this wood for the trees. The implications of this deepening understanding apply equally to new psychological and pharmacological treatment possibilities.

The second of the two Freud quotes cited above ends like this:

> [The success of a treatment for breaking addiction] will only be an apparent one, so long as the physician contents himself with withdrawing the narcotic substance from his patients, without troubling about the source from which their imperative need for it springs. . . . Whenever normal sexual life can no longer be established, we can count with certainty on the patient's relapse. [Freud, 1898a, p. 276]

This conclusion still rings true more than a century after it was first made. We would only add "social" to Freud's use of the term "sexual life", since Freud implicitly included almost all other rewarding aspects of social interaction under his broad use of the word "sexual".

Indeed, recent animal research has indicated that maternal CARE urges reduce the brain's tendency to find cocaine attractive (e.g., Ferris et al., 2005). The social attachment substitutive aspects of addiction probably go a long way to explaining why 12-step programmes are among the most effective ways to break addictive cycles. They return participants into an emotionally engaged and ultimately satisfying social network, which is so patently lacking in the lives of many addicts.

PART IV

NEUROPSYCHOANALYTIC
PERSPECTIVES ON
DREAMS

CHAPTER EIGHT

Freudian dream theory today

Mark Solms

I t is still too soon to reach a definitive verdict on the central tenets of Freud's dream theory, but recent neuropsychological research suggests that he was at least on the right track.

Summary of the theory

Freud (1900a) claimed that dreams were attempts to fulfil peremptory wishes, arising during sleep, derived from appetitive ("libidinal") urges. He based this claim on findings from a purely subjective method: he collected dreamers' associations to the individual elements of their dreams and then inferred implicit, underlying themes from the converging semantic and affective links. The "latent" thoughts revealed in this way, Freud observed, were always wishful—notwithstanding the fact that manifest dreams

---

This chapter was first published as Solms, M. (2000), "Freudian dream theory today", in *The Psychologist*, 13: 618–619.

assume a wide variety of forms, some of which appear anything but wishful.

The differences between the "manifest" and the "latent" content of dreams led Freud to infer an intervening process, by means of which the unconscious wishes could be transformed into conscious dreams. This intervening process was the so-called dream-work, which involved mechanisms such as "displacement" (substituting representational elements for one another), "condensation" (combining multiple elements into composite hybrids), and "regression" (converting thoughts into perceptions).

Why did Freud think the mind functioned in this peculiar way during sleep? He offered a cascade of hypotheses. The sleeping mind is disconnected from external reality, but not from its innate (instinctual) dispositions. These dispositions are unmodulated during sleep by the constraints of external reality. Goal-directed motor activity is impossible during sleep. The motivational programmes that are activated during sleep (and especially the peremptory ones, activated from instinctual sources) cannot be discharged in motor activity during sleep. Instead of acting on one's wishes during sleep, therefore, one imagines oneself acting on them. This imaginary (hallucinatory) fulfilment of the wish defers the pressure to act. Hence Freud's claim "that dreams are the guardians of sleep".

However, the unconstrained imaginings of the sleeping mind themselves threaten to disturb sleep (i.e., they arouse anxiety). The process of dream-work is therefore tendentiously biased in favour of more acceptable representational elements and narratives. This bias is "censorship". To the extent that the censorship fails to adequately disguise disturbing dream thoughts, the process fails and the dreamer awakens (typically from an anxiety dream).

Scientific scrutiny of the theory: first wave

In 1953, a physiological state known as "REM sleep" was discovered by Aserinsky and Kleitman. This is a paradoxical state in which one is simultaneously highly aroused and yet fast asleep. It occurs approximately every 90 minutes throughout the sleep cycle, with monotonous regularity. In 1957, Dement and Kleitman announced that dream reports were obtained from approximately

80% of awakenings from this state (Dement & Kleitman, 1957a, 1957b). By contrast, only 10% of awakenings from non-REM sleep elicited dream reports. This was the basis for the conclusion that REM sleep is the physiological equivalent of dreaming.

The brain mechanisms of REM sleep were laid bare in a succession of experiments performed mainly by Jouvet (1962) and Hobson (Hobson, McCarley, & Wyzinski, 1975): REM is switched on and off by a simple oscillatory mechanism located in a lowly part of the brainstem. This part of the brain has very little to do with mental life (its only mental function is to regulate levels of wakefulness). Accordingly, by the mid-1970s, Freud's theory was considered disproven.

Scientific scrutiny of the theory: second wave

Subsequent research revealed a more complicated state of affairs, and the simple "REM = dreaming" equation was discarded (for review, see Solms, 2000). First, Foulkes and Vogel (1965) demonstrated that far more dreams occur outside REM sleep than the early studies suggested. As many as 50% of awakenings from non-REM sleep elicit dream reports, and 20% of these are indistinguishable by any criterion from REM reports (by blind raters). Second, research by Antrobus (1991) and others revealed that the occurrence of non-REM dreams is a function of level of arousal. This suggested that the bold equation "REM = dreaming" should be replaced by a more prosaic formula: "brain activation during sleep (regardless of sleep stage) triggers dreaming". Third, it became clear that the brain mechanisms of dreaming do not coincide with those for REM sleep (Solms, 1997b, 2000).

The theoretical emphasis in the formula "brain activation during sleep triggers dreaming" falls on the word triggers. The mechanism of dreaming cannot be reduced to simple brain activation. The activation merely triggers a process that has a complex internal organization of its own. Recent research (Braun et al, 1997; Maquet et al., 1996; Nofzinger, Mintun, Wiseman, Kupfer, & Moore, 1997; Solms, 1997b) has revealed that dreams require the concerted activation of a tight network of brain mechanisms responsible for instinctual behaviours, emotion, long-term memory, and visual perception, with simultaneous deactivation of mechanisms responsible for reality monitoring and goal-directed motor activity. It appears that the instinctual and emotional mechanisms near the centre of the brain initiate the process, and that the "manifest" dream is the culmination of a process of backward projection (cf. Freud's regression) onto the perceptual structures at the back of the brain (Solms, 1997b).

These new findings are compatible with Freudian dream theory, in most respects. This is true even of Freud's central claim that dreams give expression to peremptory wishes. Dreaming is obliterated completely by damage to only two brain structures. The first of these structures forms part of a network responsible for visuospatial perception and cognition. (These are the structures that the manifest dream is "projected" onto.) It is not surprising that they should be centrally involved in dreaming. The second structure is more interesting; this is the "SEEKING" system of Panksepp (1998a), which connects the midbrain to the limbic system and frontal lobes. No single brain system comes closer in its functional properties than this one to the "libido" of Freudian dream theory. It is therefore of no small interest that among the instinctual and emotional command systems implicated in dream generation, this one seems to be pivotal (Solms, 2000). Damage to this structure results in a total cessation of dreaming (together with sharply reduced motivation) and dreams can be artificially manipulated by stimulation and inhibition of this structure, without any concomitant effect on the REM state.

In summary, it is still too soon to reach a definitive verdict on some central tenets of Freud's dream theory, but recent neuropsychological research suggests that he was at least on the right track. At minimum, the close link between brain structures responsible for dreaming, and those responsible for biological emotions and motivations, is consistent with the idea that dreams give expression to instinctual drives. The aspect of Freudian dream theory that is most difficult (although not impossible) to reconcile with current neuropsychological knowledge is that of "censorship" (for a discussion of this issue, see Hobson, 2000).

CHAPTER NINE

The Interpretation of Dreams and the neurosciences

Mark Solms

Shortly after Freud's death, the study of dreaming from the perspective of neuroscience began in earnest. Initially, these studies yielded results that were hard to reconcile with the psychological conclusions set out in *The Interpretation of Dreams* (1900a). The first major breakthrough came in 1953, when Aserinsky and Kleitman discovered a physiological state that occurs periodically

---

This chapter was first presented orally as Solms, M. (1999), "The interpretation of dreams and the neurosciences", at a Scientific Meeting of the British Psychoanalytical Society: *"The Interpretation of Dreams*: 100 Years and Many Meanings Later"*, London. It was first published as Solms, M. (1999), "The interpretation of dreams and the neurosciences", in the *British Psychoanalytical Society Bulletin*, 35 (9): 28–36; it was republished in German translation as Solms, M. (2000), "Traumdeutung und Neurowissenschaften", in J. Starobinski, I. Grubrich-Simitis, & M. Solms (Eds.), *Hundert Jahre "Traumdeutung" von Sigmund Freud: Drei Essays* (Frankfurt: Fischer), pp. 101–120 [2nd edition, 2006]; and it was republished again in a slightly revised version as Solms, M. (2001), "The interpretation of dreams and the neurosciences", in *Psychoanalysis and History*, 3: 79–91; and republished again in a further revised version as Solms, M. (2007), "*The Interpretation of Dreams* and the neurosciences", in L. Mayes, P. Fonagy, & M. Target (Eds.), *Developmental Science and Psychoanalysis: Integration and Innovation* (London: Karnac), pp. 141–158.

(in 90-minute cycles) throughout sleep, and occupies approximately 25% of our sleeping hours. This state is characterized, amongst other things, by heightened brain activation, bursts of rapid eye movement (REM), increased breathing and heart rate, genital engorgement, and paralysis of bodily movement. It consists, in short, in a paradoxical physiological condition in which one is simultaneously highly aroused and yet fast asleep. Not surprisingly, Aserinsky and Kleitman suspected that this REM state (as it came to be known) was the external manifestation of the subjective dream state. That suspicion was soon confirmed experimentally, by Aserinsky and Kleitman (1955) and Dement and Kleitman (1957a, 1957b). It is now generally accepted that if someone is awakened from REM sleep and asked whether or not he has been dreaming, he will report that he was dreaming in as many as 95% of such awakenings. Non-REM sleep, by contrast, yields dream reports at a rate of only 5–10% of awakenings.

These early discoveries generated great excitement in the neuroscientific field: for the first time it appeared to have in its grasp an objective, physical manifestation of dreaming, the most subjective of all mental states. All that remained to be done, it seemed, was to lay bare the brain mechanisms that produced this physiological state; then we would have discovered nothing less than how the brain produces dreams. Since the REM state can be demonstrated in almost all mammals, this research could also be conducted in subhuman species (which has important methodological implications, for brain mechanisms can be manipulated in animal experiments in ways that they cannot in human research).

A sequence of studies followed, in quick succession, in which different parts of the brain were systematically removed (in cats) in order to isolate the precise structures that produced REM sleep. On this basis, Jouvet was able to report in 1962 that REM (and therefore dreaming) was produced by a small region of cells in a part of the brainstem known as the "pons". This part of the nervous system is situated at a level only slightly above the spinal cord, near the nape of the neck. The higher levels of the brain, such as the cerebral hemispheres themselves which fill out the great hollow of the human skull, did not appear to play any causal role whatever in the generation of dreaming. REM sleep occurs with monotonous regularity throughout sleep, so long as the pons is intact, even if the great cerebral hemispheres are removed completely.

Neuroscientific research into the mechanism of REM sleep continued along these lines, using a wide variety of methods, and by 1975 a detailed picture of the anatomy and physiology of "dreaming sleep" had emerged. This picture, which is embodied in the *reciprocal interaction* and *activation-synthesis* models of McCarley and Hobson (1975, 1977), has dominated the field ever since—or, at least, as we shall see, until very recently. These authoritative models proposed that REM sleep and dreaming were literally "switched on" by a small group of cells situated deep within the pons, which excrete a chemical called acetylcholine. This chemical activates the higher parts of the brain, which are thereby prompted to generate (meaningless) conscious images. These meaningless images are nothing more than the higher brain making "the best of a bad job . . . from the noisy signals sent up from the brain stem" (Hobson & McCarley, 1977, p. 1347). After a few minutes of REM activity, the cholinergic activation arising from the brainstem is counteracted by another group of cells, also situated in the pons, which excrete two other chemicals: noradrenaline and serotonin. These chemicals "switch off" the cholinergic activation (and thereby, according to the theory, the conscious experience of dreaming).

Thus all the complex mental processes that Freud elucidated in *The Interpretation of Dreams* (1900a) were swept aside and replaced by a simple oscillatory mechanism by means of which consciousness is automatically switched on and off at approximately 90 minute intervals throughout sleep by reciprocally interacting chemicals that are excreted in an elementary part of the brain that has nothing to do with complex mental functions. Thus, even the most basic claims of Freud's theory no longer seemed tenable:

> The primary motivating force of dreaming is not psychological but physiological since the time of occurrence and duration of dreaming sleep are quite constant suggesting a pre-programmed, neurally determined genesis. In fact, the neural mechanisms involved can now be precisely specified. . . . If we assume that the physiological substrate of consciousness

is in the forebrain, these facts [i.e. that REM is automatically generated by brainstem mechanisms] completely eliminate any possible contribution of ideas (or their neural substrate) to the primary driving force of the dream process. [Hobson & McCarley, 1977, pp. 1346, 1338]

On this basis, it seemed justifiable to conclude that the causal mechanisms underlying dreaming were "motivationally neutral" (McCarley & Hobson, 1977, p. 1219) and that dream imagery was nothing more than "the best possible fit of intrinsically inchoate data produced by the auto-activated brain-mind" (Hobson, 1988, p. 204). The credibility of Freud's theory was, in short, severely strained by the first wave of data about dreaming that was obtained from "anatomical preparations" (Freud, 1900a, p. 536), and the neuroscientific world (indeed the scientific world as a whole) reverted to the pre-psychoanalytic view that "dreams are froth" (Freud, 1900a, p. 133).

However, alongside the observations just reviewed, which provided an increasingly precise and detailed picture of the neurology of REM sleep, a second body of evidence gradually began to accumulate, which led some neuroscientists to recognize that *perhaps REM sleep was not the physiological equivalent of dreaming after all* (Solms, 2000).

The notion that dreaming is merely "an epiphenomenon of REM sleep" (Hobson, Stickgold, & Pace-Schott, 1998, p. 12) rested almost exclusively on the observation that arousal from the REM state yielded dream reports on 70–95% of awakenings, whereas non-REM awakenings yielded such reports in only 5–10% of attempts. Considering the vagaries of subjective memory (and especially memory for dreams), this is as close to a perfect correlation as one could reasonably expect. However, the sharp division between REM ("dreaming") sleep and non-REM ("non-dreaming") sleep began to fray when it was discovered that reports of complex mentation could, in fact, be elicited in as many as 50% of awakenings from non-REM sleep. This became apparent when Foulkes awakened subjects from non-REM sleep and asked them, "What was passing through your mind?" rather than, "Have you been dreaming?" (Foulkes, 1962). The resultant non-REM dream reports were more "thought-like" (less vivid) than the REM dream reports but this distinction held only for the statistical average. The fact remained that at least 5–10% of non-REM dream reports were "indistinguishable by any criterion from those obtained from post-REM awakenings" (Hobson, 1988, p. 143). These findings "do not support a dichotomic distinction between REM and NREM mentation, rather they suggest the hypothesis of the existence of continuous dream processing characterised by a variability within and between sleep stages" (Cavallero, Cicogna, Natale, Occhionero, & Zito, 1992, p. 563).

The non-REM dream reports could not be explained away as misremembered REM dreams, for it soon became apparent that dream reports could regularly be obtained even before the dreamer had entered the first REM phase. In fact, we now know that dream reports are obtainable from as many as 50–70% of awakenings during the sleep-onset phase—that is, in the first few minutes after falling asleep (Foulkes, Spear, & Symonds, 1966; Foulkes & Vogel, 1965; Vogel, Barrowclough, & Giesler, 1972). This is a far higher rate than at any other point during the non-REM cycle, and almost as high as the REM rate. Similarly, it was recently discovered that non-REM dreams appear with increasing length and frequency towards the end of sleep, during the rising morning phase of the diurnal rhythm (Kondo, Antrobus, & Fein, 1989). In other words, non-REM dreams do not appear randomly during the sleep cycle; dreaming is generated during non-REM sleep by specific non-REM mechanisms.

The only reliable difference between REM dream reports, sleep-onset reports, and certain other classes of non-REM dream report is that the REM reports are longer. In all other respects, the non-REM and REM dreams appear to be identical. This demonstrates conclusively that fully fledged dreams can occur independently of the unique physiological state of REM sleep. Therefore, whatever the explanation may be for the strong correlation that exists between dreaming and REM sleep, it is no longer accepted that dreaming is caused exclusively by the REM state.

The presumed isomorphism between REM sleep and dreaming was further undermined by the emergence, very recently, of new and unexpected evidence regarding the brain mechanisms of dreaming. As already noted, the hypothesis that dreaming is merely an epiphenomenon of REM sleep rested on the high correlation between REM awakening and dream reports. But this does not necessarily imply that REM and dreaming share a unitary brain mechanism. In the light of the discovery that dreams regularly occur independently of REM sleep, it is certainly possible that the REM state and dreaming are controlled by independent brain mechanisms. The two mechanisms could well be situated in different parts of the brain, with the REM mechanism frequently triggering the dream mechanism. A two-stage causation of REM dreaming implies that the dream mechanism could also be stimulated into action by triggers other than the REM mechanism, which would explain why dreaming so frequently occurs outside REM sleep.

This hypothesis, that two separate mechanisms—one for REM and one for dreaming—exist in the brain, can easily be tested by a standard neurological research method known as clinico-anatomical correlation. This is the classical method for testing such hypotheses: the parts of the brain that obliterate REM sleep are removed, and the investigator observes whether or not dreaming still occurs; then the parts of the brain that obliterate dreaming are removed, and the investigator observes whether or not REM still occurs. If the two effects dissociate, then they are caused by different brain mechanisms. If they are affected simultaneously by damage to a single brain structure, then they are served by a unitary mechanism.

It is known that destruction of parts of the pons (and nowhere else) leads to a cessation of REM sleep in lower mammals (Jones, 1979), but such experiments cannot, of course, be performed on humans—the only species that is in a position to tell us whether or not destruction of those parts of the brain leads simultaneously to a cessation of dreaming. Fortunately (for science), the relevant brain structures are occasionally destroyed in human cases by naturally occurring damage, due to spontaneous illness or traumatic injury to the brain. Twenty-six such cases have been reported in the neurological literature, with damage to the pons, which resulted in a total or near-total loss of REM sleep. Surprisingly, the elimination of REM in these cases was accompanied by reported loss of dreaming in only one of the 26 patients (Feldman, 1971). In the other 25 cases, the investigators either could not establish this correlation or they did not consider it. By contrast, in all the other cases ever published in the neuroscientific literature in which damage to the brain did result in a reported loss of dreaming (a total of 110 patients), a completely different part of the brain was damaged and the pons was spared completely. Moreover, it has been proven that REM sleep is completely preserved in these cases, despite their loss of dreaming. This dissociation between cessation of REM and cessation of dreaming seriously undermines the doctrine that the REM state is the physiological equivalent of the dream state.

The parts of the brain that are crucial for dreaming and those that are crucial for REM sleep are widely separated, both anatomically and functionally. The parts of the brain that are crucial for REM are in the pons, which is located in the brainstem, near the nape of the neck. The parts of the brain that are crucial for dreaming, by contrast, are situated exclusively in the higher parts of the brain, in two specific locations within the cerebral hemispheres themselves.

The first of these locations is in the deep white matter of the frontal lobes of the brain, just above the eyes (Solms, 1997b). This part of the frontal lobes contains a large fibre-pathway, which transmits a chemical called "dopamine" from the middle of the brain to the higher parts of the brain. Damage to this pathway renders dreaming impossible but leaves the REM cycle completely unaffected (Jus et al., 1973). This suggests that dreaming is generated by a different mechanism than the one that generates REM sleep: a conclusion which is strongly supported by the observation that chemical stimulation of this dopamine pathway (with drugs like L-DOPA) leads to a massive increase in the frequency and vividness of dreams without it having any effect on the frequency and intensity of REM sleep (Hartmann, Russ, Oldfield, Falke, & Skoff, 1980; Klawans, Moskowitz, Lupton, & Scharf, 1978; Nausieda, Weiner, Kaplan, Weber, & Klawans, 1982; Scharf, Moscovitz, Lupton, & Klawans, 1978). Likewise, excessively frequent and vivid dreaming which is caused by dopamine stimulants can be stopped by drugs (like anti-psychotics) that block the transmission of dopamine in this pathway (Sacks, 1985, 1990, 1991). In short, dreaming can be switched "on" and "off" by a neurochemical pathway that has nothing to do with the REM oscillator in the pons. What, then, is the function of this higher brain pathway which is so crucial for the generation of dreams? Its main function is to "instigate goal-seeking behaviors and an organism's appetitive interactions with the world" (Panksepp, 1985, p. 273)—that is, to motivate the subject to seek out and engage with external objects that can satisfy its inner biological needs. These are precisely the functions that Freud attributed to the "libidinal drive"—the primary instigator of dreams—in his (1900a) theory. Accordingly, it is of considerable interest to note that damage to this pathway causes cessation of dreaming in conjunction with a massive reduction in motivated behaviour (Solms, 1997b). In view of the close association between dreams and certain forms of insanity, it is also interesting to note that surgical damage to this pathway (which was the primary target of the prefrontal leucotomies of the 1950s and 1960s) leads to a reduction in some symptoms of psychotic illness, together with a cessation of dreaming (Frank, 1946, 1950; Partridge, 1950; Schindler, 1953). Whatever it is that prevented leucotomized patients from maintaining their psychiatric symptoms also prevented them from generating dreams.

In short, the current neuroscientific evidence gives us every reason to take seriously the radical hypothesis—first set out by Freud a 100 years ago—to the effect that dreams are motivated phenomena, driven by our wishes. Although it is true that the (cholinergic) mechanism that generates the REM state is "motivationally neutral", this cannot be said of the (dopaminergic) mechanism that generates the dream state. In fact, the latter mechanism is the appetitive (i.e., libidinal) "command system" of the brain (Panksepp, 1985, 1998a).

As stated, it now appears that REM only causes dreaming via the intermediary of this motivational mechanism. Moreover, REM is just one of the many different triggers that are capable of activating this mechanism. A variety of other triggers, which act independently of REM, have exactly the same effect. Sleep-onset dreams and late-morning dreams are two examples of this kind. Dreams induced by L-DOPA (and various stimulant drugs) are further examples. Of special interest in this regard is the fact that recurring, stereotyped nightmares can be induced by seizures that occur during sleep. We know from the work of Penfield[1] exactly where in the brain these seizures begin—namely, in the temporal limbic system. This system, which subserves emotional and memory functions, is situated in the higher forebrain and is richly interconnected with the frontal-lobe dopamine pathway discussed above. Moreover, we know that such seizures usually occur during non-REM sleep

(Janz, 1974; Kellaway & Frost, 1983). The fact that nightmares can be "switched on" by mechanisms in the higher parts of the brain which have nothing to do with the pons and nothing to do with REM sleep is further evidence that dreaming and REM are generated by separate and independent brain mechanisms.

It is surely no accident that what all of these different mechanisms capable of triggering dreams have in common is the fact that they create a state of arousal during sleep. This lends support to another of the cardinal hypotheses that Freud put forward in this book—namely, the hypothesis that dreams are a response to something that disturbs sleep.[2] But it appears that the arousal stimuli enumerated above only trigger dreaming if and when they activate the final common motivational pathway within the frontal lobes of the brain, for it is only when this pathway is removed (rather than the arousal triggers themselves, including REM) that dreaming becomes impossible. This relationship between the various arousal triggers and the dream-onset mechanism itself is reminiscent of Freud's famous analogy: dreaming only occurs if the stimulus that acts as the "entrepreneur" of the dream attracts the support of a "capitalist", an unconscious libidinal urge, which alone has the power to generate dreaming (1900a, p. 561).

Thus, Freud's major inferences from psychological evidence regarding both the causes and the function of dreaming are at least compatible with, and even indirectly supported by, current neuroscientific knowledge. Does the same apply to the mechanism of dreaming?

Our current neuroscientific understanding of the mechanism of dreaming revolves centrally around the concept of regression. The prevailing view is that imagery of all kinds (including dream imagery) is generated by "projecting information backward in the system" (Kosslyn, 1994, p. 75). Accordingly, dreaming is conceptualized as "internally generated images which are fed backwards into the cortex as if they were coming from the outside" (Zeki, 1993, p. 326). This conception of dream imagery is based on wide-ranging neurophysiological and neuropsychological research into numerous aspects of visual processing. However, the regressive nature of dream processing has recently been demonstrated directly in clinical neurological cases (Solms, 1997b).

In order to illustrate this point, it is necessary to remind the reader that loss of dreaming due to neurological damage is associated with damage in two brain locations. The first of these is the white-fibre pathway of the frontal lobes, which we have considered already. The second location is a portion of the grey cortex at the back of the brain (just behind and above the ears) called the occipito-temporo-parietal junction. This part of the brain performs the highest levels of processing of perceptual information, and it is essential for:

> the conversion of concrete perception into abstract thinking, which always proceeds in the form of internal schemes, and for the memorizing of organized experience or, in other words, not only for the perception of information but also for its storage. [Luria, 1973, p. 74]

The fact that dreaming ceases completely with damage to this part of the brain suggests that these functions (the conversion of concrete perceptions into abstract thoughts and memories), like the motivational functions performed by the frontal-lobe pathway discussed previously, are fundamental to the whole process of dreaming. However, if the theory that dream imagery is generated by a process that reverses the normal sequence of events in perceptual processing is correct, then we may expect that, in dreams, abstract thoughts and memories are converted into concrete perceptions. This is exactly what Freud had in mind when he wrote that, "in regression, the fabric of the dream-thoughts is resolved into its raw material" (1900a, p. 543). This inference is supported empirically by the observation that dreaming as a whole stops completely with damage at the highest level of the perceptual systems (in the region of the occipito-temporo-junction), whereas only specific aspects of dream imagery are affected by damage at lower levels of the visual system, closer to the perceptual periphery (in the region of the occipital lobe). This implies that the contribution of the higher levels precedes that of the lower levels. When there is damage at the higher levels, dreaming is blocked completely, whereas damage at the lower levels merely subtracts something from the terminal stage of the dream process. This is the opposite of what happens in waking perception, which is obliterated entirely by damage at the lowest levels of the system. In other words, dreaming reverses the normal sequence of perceptual events.

The available neuroscientific evidence, therefore, is compatible with Freud's conception of where and how the dream process is initiated (e.g., by an arousing stimulus that activates the emotional and motivational systems) and of where and how it terminates (such as by abstract thinking in the memory systems, which is projected backwards in the form of concrete images onto the perceptual systems).

In fact, it is now possible to actually *see* where this neural activity is distributed in the dreaming brain. Modern neuroradiological methods produce pictures of the pattern of metabolic activity in the living brain while it is actually performing a particular function, and in the case of dreaming these images clearly show how the brain's energic "cathexis" (as Freud called it) is concentrated within the anatomical areas discussed above—namely, the (frontal and limbic) parts of the brain concerned with arousal, emotion, memory, and motivation, on the one hand, and the parts (at the back of the brain) concerned with abstract thinking and visual perception, on the other.

These radiological pictures also reveal something about what happens in between the initial and terminal ends of the dream process. The most striking feature of the dreaming brain in this respect is the fact that a region of the brain known as the dorsolateral frontal convexity is completely inactive during dreams. This is striking, because this part of the brain, which is inactive during dreams, is one of the most active of all brain areas during waking mental activity. If one compares the pictures of the waking brain with those of the dreaming brain, one literally sees the truth of Fechner's (1889) assertion to the effect that "the scene of action of dreams is different from that of waking ideational life" (cf. Freud, 1900a, p. 536). Whereas in waking ideational life, the "scene of action" is concentrated in the dorsolateral region at the front of the brain—"the upper end of the motor system—the gateway from thought to action" (Solms, 1997b, p. 223)—in dreams it is concentrated in the occipito-temporo-parietal region at the back of the brain, on the memory and perceptual systems. In short, in dreams, the "scene" shifts from the motor end of the apparatus to the perceptual end.[3] This reflects the fact that whereas in waking life the normal course of mental events is directed toward action, in dreams this path is unavailable. The "gateway" to the motor systems (the dorsolateral frontal convexity of the brain) is blocked in dreams (Braun et al., 1997, 1998; Solms, 1997b), as are the motor output channels (the alpha motor neurons of the spinal cord; Pompeiano, 1979). Thus both the intention to act and the ability to act are blocked during sleep, and it seems reasonable to infer (as did Freud) that this block is the immediate cause of the dream process assuming a regressive path, away from the motor systems of the brain, toward the perceptual systems (Solms, 1997b).

Finally, due to relative inactivation during sleep of crucial parts of the reflective systems in the frontal parts of the limbic brain, the imagined dream scene is uncritically accepted and the dreamer mistakes the internally generated scene for a real perception. Damage to these reflective systems (which evidently are not entirely inactive during sleep) results in a curious state of almost constant dreaming during sleep and an inability to distinguish between thoughts and real events during waking life. This provides further evidence of a continuous thought process occurring during sleep, which is converted into dreaming under various physiological conditions, of which REM sleep is just one among many.

The picture of the dreaming brain which emerges from recent neuroscientific research may therefore be summarized as follows: the process of dreaming is initiated by an arousal stimulus. If this stimulus is sufficiently intense or persistent to activate the motivational mechanisms of the brain (or if it attracts the interest of these mechanisms for some other reason), the dream process proper begins. The functioning of the motivational systems of the brain is normally channelled towards goal-directed action, but access to the motor systems is blocked during sleep. The purposive action that would be the normal outcome of motivated interest is thereby rendered impossible during sleep. As a result (and quite possibly in order to protect sleep), the process of activation assumes a regressive course. This appears to involve a two-stage process. First, the higher parts of the perceptual systems (which serve memory and abstract thinking) are activated; then the lower parts (which serve concrete imagery) are activated. As a result of this regressive process, the dreamer does not actually engage in motivated activity during sleep, but, rather, imagines himself to be doing so. Due to inactivation during sleep of the reflective systems in the frontal part of the limbic brain, the imagined scene is uncritically accepted, and the dreamer mistakes it for a real perception.

There is a great deal about the dreaming brain that we still do not understand. It is also evident that we have not yet discovered the neurological correlates of some crucial components of the "dream-work" as Freud understood it. The function of "censorship" is the most glaring example of this kind. However, we are beginning to understand something about the neurological correlates of that function, and we know at least that the structures that are most likely to be implicated (Solms, 1998b) are indeed highly active during dreaming sleep (Braun et al., 1997, 1998).

Hopefully it is apparent to the reader from this brief overview that the picture of the dreaming brain which has begun to emerge from the most recent neuroscientific researches is broadly compatible with the psychological theory that Freud advanced. In fact, aspects of Freud's account of the dreaming mind are so consistent with the currently available neuroscientific data that I personally think we would be well advised to use Freud's model as a guide for the next phase of our neuroscientific investigations. Unlike the research effort of the past few decades, the next stage in our search for the brain mechanisms of dreaming (if it is to succeed) must take as its starting point the new perspective we have gained on the role of REM sleep. REM sleep, which has hitherto diverted our attention away from the neuropsychological mechanisms of dreaming, should simply be added to the various "somatic sources" of dreams that Freud discussed in chapters 1 and 5 of his book (1900a). The major focus of our future research efforts should then be directed towards elucidating the brain correlates of the mechanisms that Freud discussed in his sixth and seventh chapters: the mechanisms of the dream-work proper:

> We shall feel no surprise at the over-estimation of the part played in forming dreams by stimuli which do not arise from mental life. Not only are they easy to discover and even open to experimental confirmation; but the somatic view of the origin of dreams is completely in line with the prevailing trend of thought in psychiatry to-day. It is true that the dominance of the brain over the organism is asserted with apparent confidence.

Nevertheless, anything that might indicate that mental life is in any way independent of demonstrable organic changes or that its manifestations are in any way spontaneous alarms the modern psychiatrist, as though a recognition of such things would inevitably bring back the days of the Philosophy of Nature, and the metaphysical view of the nature of mind. The suspicions of the psychiatrists have put the mind, as it were, under tutelage, and they now insist that none of its impulses shall be allowed to suggest that it has any means of its own. This behaviour of theirs only shows how little trust they really have in the validity of a causal connection between the somatic and the mental. Even when investigation shows the primary exciting cause of a phenomenon is psychical, deeper research will one day trace the path further and discover an organic basis for the mental event. But if at the moment we cannot see beyond the mental, that is no reason for denying its existence. [Freud, 1900a, pp. 41–42]

Notes

1. Penfield was able to artificially generate the recurring nightmare scenes by directly stimulating the seizure focus in the temporal lobe (Penfield, 1938; Penfield & Erickson, 1941; Penfield & Rasmussen, 1950).

2. Solms (1995, 1997b) provides limited empirical evidence to support the hypothesis that dreams protect sleep: patients who lose the ability to dream due to brain damage report more disturbed sleep than brain damaged patients with intact dreaming.

3. It is of utmost interest to note that the major inhibitory systems of the forebrain are concentrated at its motor end, as they were in Freud's (1900a) diagrammatic representation of the mental apparatus.

PART V

NEUROPSYCHOANALYTIC PERSPECTIVES ON CONSCIOUSNESS

CHAPTER TEN

The "id" knows more than the "ego" admits

Mark Solms & Jaak Panksepp

1. Introduction

Our aim here is to introduce a novel way of integrating affective and cognitive aspects of conscious and unconscious brain processes, using a neuropsychoanalytic framework. Our starting point is the commonplace observation that different fields of inquiry use the terms "conscious" and "unconscious" in different ways, which prevents coherent discourse among the disciplines. The field at large has no standard definitions of these terms and their cognates. For instance, what is conscious "awareness"? Does the conscious subject need to have more than simple phenomenal experiences to have conscious "awareness"? Does "awareness" always imply a capacity for reflexive recognition of

This chapter was first presented orally as Solms, M. (2011), "The conscious id", at a scientific meeting of the Arnold Pfeffer Center for Neuropsychoanalysis at the New York Psychoanalytic Institute; it was presented again in many other forums thereafter in substantially different versions. It was first published as Solms, M., & Panksepp, J. (2012), "The 'id' knows more than the 'ego' admits", in *Brain Sciences*, 2: 147–175; and it was republished in a substantially revised version as Solms, M. (2013), "The conscious id", in *Neuropsychoanalysis*, 15: 5–85.

the fact that one is having experiences? Can we have (and empirically study) phenomenal consciousness without higher forms of consciousness that can report about awareness? We believe the answer to the last question has to be "yes"; otherwise we exclude all other animals from the circle of consciousness, which makes no evolutionary sense, especially given the abundant evidence for "rewarding" and "punishing" brain functions concentrated in various subcortical brainstem regions.

To avoid such ambiguities, we start from the premise that the essential nature of consciousness is a foundational form of phenomenal experience, which in our view includes various affective states that can be monitored in animals by the rewarding and punishing properties of artificial evocation of such states with deep brain stimulation. From our perspective, the capacity to be aware of the environment and that one is the subject of such externally triggered experiences is already a higher cognitive function, which is ultimately mediated by the ability to reflect upon one's subjective experiences. This hierarchical parsing enables one to be conscious in different ways—for example, to feel happy and sad, without necessarily having the mental capacity to recognize that one is happy or sad, let alone to reflect upon the objective relations that caused this happiness or sadness. Being phenomenally conscious does not, by itself, require much cognitive sophistication at all.

2.   Synopsis of our overall framework

Such modest conceptual distinctions permit the construction of evolutionarily sound scientific approaches to consciousness, which enable us, for example, to distinguish the brain structures supporting its phylogenetically ancient forms—which, based on abundant empirical studies, are affectively shared by all mammals—from those supporting the higher forms of consciousness that require reflexive and declarative abilities, which can only be studied systematically in creatures that speak for themselves. Failure to make such distinctions produces types of discourse that prematurely render lower brain processes "unconscious" simply because the forms of internally generated experiences are not often recognized, and easily spoken about, by higher, specifically human forms of linguistically based awareness. For example, certain mammalian species may have a great abundance of affectively and perceptually conscious phenomenal experiences, with very little capacity to reflect on those experiences. An evolutionarily tiered approach to consciousness also allows us to understand how it happens that strong affective states can occur without the subject of those states cognitively recognizing ("accepting") the associated feelings. Moreover, since higher functions can inhibit lower functions in the brain (and *vice-versa*), we can see how certain forms of phenomenal experience may be temporarily rendered "unconscious" through active inhibitory influences. Strong emotions can also interfere with and disrupt cognitive processing, so it readily happens that individuals may experience strong emotional turmoil without having any subsequent insight into, or even memory of, those experiences. These examples could easily be multiplied.

In short, the complexity of our capacity to consciously and unconsciously process fluctuating brain states and environmentally linked behavioural processes requires some kind of multi-tiered analysis, such as Endel Tulving's well-known parsing of consciousness into three forms: *anoetic* (unthinking forms of experience, which may be affectively intense without being "known" and could be the birthright of all mammals), *noetic* (thinking forms of consciousness, linked to exteroceptive perception and cognition) and *autonoetic* (abstracted forms of perceptions and cognitions, which allow conscious "awareness" and reflection upon experience in the "mind's eye" through episodic memories and fantasies) (Tulving, 2002).

This kind of a conceptual scheme can be readily overlaid on some major evolutionary passages of the brain, which roughly correspond to the evolution of (a) upper brainstem (up to the septal area), which permits *anoetic* phenomenal experiences, (b) lower subcortical ganglia and upper limbic structures (e.g., the cortical midline), which permit learning and *noetic* consciousness, and (c) higher neocortical functions (including all association cortices), which provide the critical substrates for the *autonoetic*, reflexive experiential blends that yield the stream of everyday awareness. Such multi-tiered parsing of consciousness (see Figure 10.1) enables us to recognize not only deeply unconscious brain processes, critical

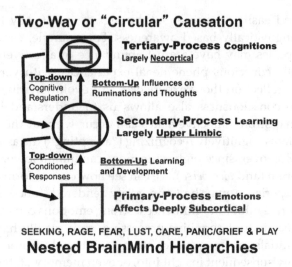

Two-Way or "Circular" Causation

Tertiary-Process Cognitions
Largely <u>Neocortical</u>

Top-down
Cognitive
Regulation

Bottom-Up Influences on
Ruminations and Thoughts

Secondary-Process Learning
Largely <u>Upper Limbic</u>

Top-down
Conditioned
Responses

Bottom-Up Learning
and Development

Primary-Process Emotions
Affects Deeply <u>Subcortical</u>

SEEKING, RAGE, FEAR, LUST, CARE, PANIC/GRIEF & PLAY

Nested BrainMind Hierarchies

FIGURE 10.1.   A schematic showing nested hierarchies of brain functions in which primary processes (red squares) influence secondary (green circles) and tertiary (blue rectangles) processes, which in turn exert top-down regulatory control. The seven primary process emotions are noted: positively valenced emotions highlighted in red (SEEKING, LUST, CARE and PLAY), and negative ones in purple (RAGE, FEAR and PANIC/GRIEF) (adapted from Panksepp, 1998a, 2011).

for behaviour, but also brain processes that may be experienced at one level but not at another. This permits us to include in our scientific discourse the massive and ever-mounting evidence for the existence of various perceptual and affective forms of phenomenal consciousness in other animals (Merker, 2007; Panksepp, 1998a). This may enable us to develop better neuroevolutionary paradigms to scientifically unravel the fundamental biological nature of consciousness, as well as the differential natures of its many strange manifestations across multiple levels.

Here we will address the multi-tiered complexities of consciousness from both modern cognitive and affective-neuroscience perspectives. However, to properly contextualize these perspectives historically, we will frame selected aspects of the cognitive and affective data within a psychoanalytic frame of reference, which remains surprisingly relevant for the controversies under discussion here. Although the interregnum of "never-mind" behaviourism, which simply ignored the Black Box of the brain, interrupts the historical continuities, we hope that embedding our discussion in a clear account of seminal foundational issues that were explicitly considered at the outset of the modern neuroscientific era will help us better understand what the splintered subfields of current neuroscience can and must still achieve. Our hope is that this will eventually yield a unified vision of how the mind actually works.

To set the stage in a historical perspective, we contextualize our argument within the theoretical framework of classic psychoanalytic thought that may help highlight some provocative conceptual relationships to our approach. A close reading of Freudian thought suggests that he took a very similar approach to the mind. Even though Freud, a bench neuroscientist at the beginning of his career, did not have the wealth of neuroscientific knowledge we presently have, our objective analysis of the mental apparatus has distinct resemblances to his efforts, which emerged strictly from the subjective perspective. We offer this as an example of convergence, which hopefully promotes more careful empirical analyses of the affective foundations of the human mind than have been evident in so much of modern neuroscience, which typically offers a ruthlessly reductionistic view of the brain, as if an analysis of the mental apparatus is irrelevant for understanding what the brain does.

3.   Freud's notion of unconscious mental processes

The notion that the brain knows more than it consciously admits can be traced back historically to the clinical and conceptual work of Sigmund Freud. He based this notion, which was considered radical at the time, upon observations he made of post-hypnotic suggestion and clinical states of dissociation, where behaviours were demonstrably caused by motivations of which the subject was not explicitly aware, some of which could subsequently be brought to awareness during psychological treatment. Since a scientific account of mental life cannot exclude unconscious cognitions with such demonstrable causal effects, Freud concluded that the objects of psychology must include unconscious processes, notwithstanding the conventional equation of "mind" with consciousness (Freud, 1915e). Thus, Freud devoted the remainder of his scientific life to studying the unconscious mental processes.

His first major conclusion was that such processes admitted of further differentiation. Some unconscious processes could be rendered conscious at will; others could not. Freud termed these processes "preconscious" and "unconscious", respectively. He then subdivided the unconscious processes into those that occurred outside conscious awareness by dint of automatization (e.g., habituated skills) and those that were actively excluded from awareness by motivated resistances (e.g., electing not to think about something in order to avoid negative affective arousal). He termed these processes "descriptively" and "dynamically" unconscious, respectively. The dynamically unconscious processes included some that were "repressed" from consciousness and some that never attained consciousness in the first place.

Freud's second major conclusion was that these different grades of unconscious process displayed different functional properties. Dynamically unconscious processes were less constrained by realistic life considerations than were preconscious or descriptively unconscious ones. The latter processes were, conversely, less influenced by affective states than were the dynamically unconscious ones. On this basis, Freud differentiated mental processes that obeyed what he termed the "reality principle" from those that obeyed the "pleasure principle", with the latter being relatively unconstrained by inhibitory controls. In modern terms, they may be conceptualized as being activated by "free energy" (Bernroider & Panksepp, 2011; Kiebel & Friston, 2011). Since the uninhibited processes were assumed to be phylogenetically older, and predominated in the juvenile mind, Freud termed them "primary"; the inhibited, realistic processes were described as "secondary" (which in Figure 10.1 are further distinguished into secondary—namely, learned—and tertiary—namely, thought-related—processes).

Borrowing from Helmholtzian thermodynamics (Helmholtz, 1886), Freud speculated that secondary processes[1] entail some form of "binding" of "free" energies, arising from the vital needs of the organism, although he admitted his ignorance of the underlying physiology of these processes. He inferred that the compulsive "free" energies press for immediate motor discharge (since they are unconstrained by realistic considerations), whereas "bound" energies, which are utilized in executive cognitive processes, give rise to more expedient, delayed responses. Freud imagined that such hypothetical energies "spread over the memory-traces of ideas somewhat as an electric charge is spread over the surface of a body" (Freud, 1894a, p. 60). Mental processes were therefore fundamentally conceptualized by Freud as being composed of (a) representations, activated by (b) drive energies (which he sometimes also called "quotas of affect"). These two mental elements were considered to be unconscious in themselves and only to give rise to the phenomena of consciousness under certain conditions.

We will develop the theme here that these two elements remain the foundational concepts of modern cognitive and affective science, but we will argue that the so-called "drive energies" that activate cognition are intrinsically conscious—although the transformations they are subject to frequently render them inaccessible to reflexive awareness.

Freud formulated the conditional foundations of consciousness within a series of models of the functional architecture of the mind. In his first model (1950 [1895]) he attributed (unconscious) representational processes to a system of forebrain neurons that were distinguished from other neurons by their capacity for memory. He called this representational system "ψ". Freud described this system as a "sympathetic ganglion" because its biological purpose was to associatively link endogenous needs (expressed as drives) with the external objects that satisfied them. The ψ system of neurons was split into "pallium" and "nuclear" divisions. The pallium division received its inputs via subcortical thalamic and cranial-nerve pathways from the sensory periphery (Freud called these pathways the "φ" system of neurons). The nuclear division of ψ received its inputs from the interior of the body, which Freud described as the "wellspring" of the mental apparatus, for the reason that it was constantly activated (or "cathected," to use his term) by drive energies emanating from the relentless vital (survival and sexual) needs of the body. Tonic inhibition of this interoceptive division of ψ was accordingly assumed to be the physiological basis of executive control (the "ego").

Consciousness, which was attributed to a separate neuronal system ("ω"), was located at the motor end of the apparatus. The distinctive function of the ω system was to monitor the accumulation of drive energies within ψ. Increased drive tension generated feelings of unpleasure in ω; motor discharge, by contrast, generated pleasure. This affective-homeostatic function was, according to Freud, the primary purpose of consciousness. He therefore always insisted that affects were conscious by definition (see Section 11 below). Affect was the *raison d'être* of consciousness. However, consciousness was also extended to external sensory perception, by complicated mechanisms that revolved around the function of attention, which increased the level of activation of the extero-ceptive division of ψ (1925a [1924]).[2] Consciousness accordingly occurred in two forms: (a) the form attached to interoceptive affects, and (b) the form attached to exteroceptive perceptions. Regarding the qualitative differences in the forms of consciousness, Freud stated only that the various modalities appeared to arise from different rhythms or patterns or "periods" (as opposed to degrees) of neuronal activity—which at that time was an inferred process, since organized neuronal activity had not yet been measured.

Freud's second model of the mental apparatus (1900a) was essentially the same as his first, apart from the fact that the hypo-thetical neuronal systems were now given purely functional designations. This acknowledged Freud's ignorance of the anatomy and physiology of the arrangements he had described, inferred as they were from psychological and behavioural rather than neu-roscientific observations. Accordingly, the φ neurons became the "perceptual system" of the mind (abbreviated "*Pcpt.*"); the ψ neu-rons became "mnemic systems," split into uninhibited and inhib-ited divisions, which thereby became the systems "unconscious" ("*Ucs.*") and "preconscious" ("*Pcs.*") respectively (see Figure 10.2);[3] while the ω neurons became the system "consciousness" ("*Cs.*"), still located at the motor end of the apparatus.

A significant revision was introduced in 1917 when Freud (1917d [1915]) combined φ and ω (the perceptual and motor systems adja-cent to ψ) into a single integrated system for perceptual conscious-ness ("*Pcpt.–Cs.*"), on the grounds that all varieties of consciousness were at bottom perceptual. What distinguished the systems *Pcpt.* and *Cs.* was merely the sources of their stimuli and the modalities of perception they gave rise to. The classical sensory modalities, which registered the state of the outside world, were perceived on the "external surface" of the system *Pcpt.–Cs.*, while affects, which registered the state of the apparatus itself, were perceived on the "internal surface" of this same, integrated system.

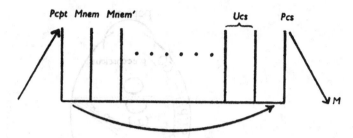

FIGURE 10.2.   Freud's second model of the mental apparatus. *Pcpt.* (previously φ) = Perceptual system; Mnem (previously ψ) = Mnemic systems; *Ucs.* = Unconscious system; *Pcs* = Preconscious system; M = Motor system [also known as the Consciousness system, abbreviated *Cs.* (previously ω)]. (Reproduced from Freud, 1915e, with permission.)

This revision was retained in Freud's final model (1923b). The major purpose of his last revision was to recognize the fact that executive control did not coincide with any grade of consciousness (or preconsciousness). For example, automatized "descriptively" unconscious processes, which never became conscious, were under inhibitory control (they were secondary processes; cf. Freud, 1915e) and served the functional purposes of the reality principle. Likewise, the process of repression, despite being "dynamically" unconscious, served inhibitory purposes. Freud thus grouped all the inhibited grades of both conscious and unconscious processes under a single executive system—the "ego"—the distinguishing feature of which was its utilization of "bound" energies (which underpinned all "cognitive" processes), and he likewise grouped all the uninhibited ("instinctual" affective) processes under a single system utilizing "free" drive energy—the "id" (see Figure 10.3).

By the end of Freud's scientific life, therefore, the notion that "the brain knows more than it admits" revolved around the theory that bottom-up interoceptive pressures on the mind produced a set of primitive, compulsive drives (in the "id") which aimed at immediate instinctual satisfaction, on the basis of affective-homeostatic imperatives regardless of the variable dictates of reality. Access by these influences to the executive motor system therefore had to be constrained, through top-down exteroceptive ("ego") influences, perception, and learning.

These theoretical developments, which introduced the very idea of unconscious mental processes to psychology, took place between

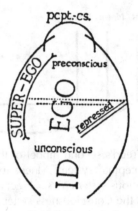

FIGURE 10.3.   Freud's final model of the mental apparatus. *Pcpt.-Cs.* = Perceptual-Consciousness system. (Reproduced from Freud, 1923b with permission.)

1894 and 1923. It is important to note that, as Freud shifted from a neurological to a functional description, his successive models of the mind still remained tethered to the body at three cardinal points: (a) the sense organs, (b) the vital needs, and (c) the motor system. Now, a century later, due to dramatic advances in the neurosciences, we are able to translate Freud's functional descriptions of these bodily origins of the mind back into the language of anatomy and physiology. We do so in Section 5 below, in the spirit of Eric Kandel's remark to the effect that Freud's models still provide "the most coherent and intellectually satisfying view of the mind" that we have (Kandel, 1999, p. 505).

4. A related modern conversation: there are two bodily origins of the mind, and they are represented differently

At the 12th International Neuropsychoanalysis Congress, held in Berlin in June 2011, on the topic of "Minding the Body", Bud Craig, Antonio Damasio, Jaak Panksepp, Vittorio Gallese, and Manos Tsakiris, among others, summarized the current state of knowledge as to how human mental functioning is embodied. In his closing remarks to the congress, Mark Solms pointed out that the speakers had referred to two different aspects of the body, without always distinguishing between them. This can lead to confusion.

The first aspect of the body pivots around somatotopic maps on the cortical surface that are derived from sensory receptors on the surface of the body. This aspect of body representation corresponds most directly to the cortical homunculus. However, it does not coincide with somatosensory cortex alone. It also includes the projection zones of the other sensory modalities, which consist of topological maps of different sensory organs. It includes also the subcortical modality-specific thalamic and cranial nerve structures that link these terminal sense organs with the cortex.

The "body image" arises not in but, rather, from these modality-specific cortical maps. This aspect of bodily representation should therefore be equated also with the various perceptual streams arising from the projection zones and converging in association cortex. In this chapter, we will call this aspect of bodily representation the "external body" for short (see Figure 10.4).

It is important to note that the brain mechanisms that represent the external body also represent other external objects. The external body is an object. It is the aspect of the body that one perceives when one looks outwards, at a mirror, for example. ("That thing is me"; it is "my body".)

It should be remembered that motor maps, too, contribute to the external body image. The sense of possessing a three-dimensional body is determined not only by heteromodal sensory convergence, but also by movement. Movement produces kinaesthetic sensations and may have intrinsic brain feelings of its own. The close relationship between movement and (muscle and joint) sensation is reflected in the anatomical proximity of the respective cortical zones: the somatosensory and motor projection areas form an integrated functional unit.

The second aspect of the body is its internal milieu, the autonomic body, which is represented deeper and lower in the brain. The brain structures that represent this aspect of the body pivot around the hypothalamus, but they also include the circumventricular organs, parabrachial nucleus, area postrema, solitary nucleus, and the like (for reviews see Damasio, 1999b, 2010; Mesulam, 2000). Analogous to what we said above about the motor cortex in relation to exteroception, these interoceptive structures, too, not only

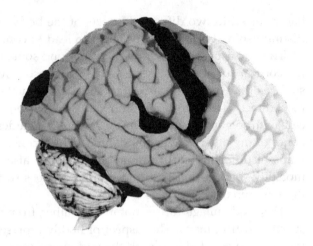

FIGURE 10.4. The external body. Dark blue = exteroceptive projection cortex; light blue = perceptual association cortex; green = motor projection cortex; yellow = motor association (executive) cortex.

monitor but also regulate the state of the body (cf. homeostasis). Such subcortical network arousals may have phenomenal affective feelings of their own. In the present chapter we will call this aspect of bodily representation the "internal body" for short (see Figure 10.5).

Even at the level of the brainstem, the neural structures for the internal body are covered by those for the external body, just as the musculoskeletal body itself envelops the viscera. This largely reflects the fact that the evolution of coherent cerebral visceration is more ancient and foundational than ambulant movement for the somatic action apparatus. There is enormous evidence that primary-process emotional action coherence, and the raw feelings that concurrently emerge, arise from these subcortical circuits (Panksepp, 1998a).

The brain mechanisms of the internal body function largely automatically, but they also arouse the external body to serve its vital needs in the external world. This is achieved through a network of upper brainstem and basal forebrain "arousal" structures known conventionally, but somewhat misleadingly, as the extended reticulo-thalamic activating system (ERTAS). This arousal system is constituted of many distinct long-axoned neuronal subsystems that include acetylcholine, epinephrine/norepinephrine, dopamine, and serotonin systems, as well as a variety of neuropeptides (Panksepp, 1998a; Pfaff, 2006). In addition, there is a complex internal structure to cerebral visceration processes (for overview see Holstege & Saper, 2005; Morgane & Panksepp, 1980; Nieuwenhuys, Voogd, & van Huijzen, 2008). The primal roots of emotionality are grounded in these autonomic substrates.

It is important to note that an interdependent, hierarchical relationship therefore exists between the two aspects of the body. Considering the evolutionarily ancient roots of visceration, situated as they are more caudally and medially in the brain, there are reasons to believe that cerebral visceration (and hence emotionality) provided a bodily coherence-generating substrate for future brain developments, including the more cognitive domains. However, as some forward-looking scholars have long emphasized, from David Hume to Antonio Damasio, the emotional components are still critically important for the way the cognitive overlay operates.

Furthermore, it is becoming ever more evident that the internal body generates a very different type of consciousness from the consciousness associated with exteroceptive cortex. The interoceptive brainstem, along with diverse emotional networks, generates

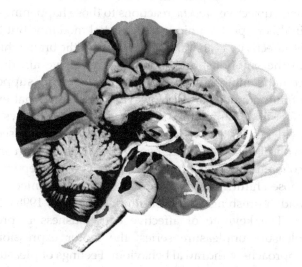

FIGURE 10.5.   The internal body. Red = some interoceptive nuclei; magenta = some ERTAS (arousal) nuclei; white = some basic emotion circuits.

internal "states" rather than external "objects" of consciousness (for reviews see Damasio, 2010; Panksepp, 1998a). In other words, the internal body is not represented as an object of perception. Rather, it gives rise to a background state of "being"; this aspect of the body is the *subject* of perception. We may picture this type of consciousness as the neurodynamic page upon which, or from which, exteroceptive experiences are written in higher brain regions. (This is also what binds experiences together; perception happens to a unitary, embodied subject; cf. the binding problem.)

It is important to note that these "states" of the body-as-subject involve not only varying levels of consciousness (e.g., sleep/waking) but also varying qualities of consciousness. Interoceptive consciousness, too, is phenomenal; it "feels like" something. Above all, the phenomenal states of the body-as-subject are experienced affectively. Affects, rather than representing discrete external events, are experienced as positively and negatively valenced states. Their valence is determined by how changing internal conditions relate to the probability of survival and reproductive success. At this level of the brain, therefore, homeostasis is inseparable from consciousness. Whereas the classical sensory modalities represent discrete external (knowledge-generating and objective) *noetic* happenings, affective consciousness represents diffuse internal (automatically evaluative and subjective) *anoetic* reactions to those happenings. Affectivity is, in this respect, a unique experiential modality. But that is not all it is; affectivity is an intrinsic property of the brain which is expressed in the emotions, and emotions are, above all, distinct forms of somatic motor discharge coordinated with supportive patterns of autonomic change. However, these emotional expressions also "feel like" something, in diversely valenced ways. The empirical evidence for the feeling component are simply based on the highly replicable fact that wherever in the brain one can artificially evoke coherent emotional response patterns with deep brain stimulation, those shifting states uniformly are accompanied by "rewarding" and "punishing" states of mind (Panksepp, 1998a, 2011).

The keynote of affective consciousness is provided by the pleasure–unpleasure series, the motor expression of which is approach–withdrawal behaviour. Feelings of pleasure–unpleasure, delight–distress—and the associated compulsive behaviours—are readily generated by stimulating as low in the brainstem as the

PAG. The generating of such reactions is thought to be the biological "purpose" of consciousness (Damasion, 1999b; Panksepp, 1998a). By attributing valence to experience—determining whether something is "good" or "bad" for the subject, within a biological system of values—affective consciousness (and the behaviours it gives rise to) intrinsically promotes survival and reproductive success. This is what consciousness is for. It also motivates the cognitive controls that emerged during further encephalization. This provides increasingly sophisticated mental strategies for controlling behaviour on the basis of what animals can do with external *noetic* information-processing.

To this end, arising from the PAG and ascending into the limbic forebrain, which reciprocally provides many descending controls, are various instinctual motivational circuits. These are also known as the circuits for "basic emotion". There are several classifications of these emotions. The best-known examples are those that generate (a) appetitive foraging, (b) consummatory reward, (c) freezing and flight, (d) aggressive attack, (e) nurturant care, (f) separation distress, and (g) rough-and-tumble play (for detailed review see Panksepp, 1998a). The circuits for these basic emotions have been given special names (see below). Further analysis of their trajectories, neurochemistries, and neurodynamics provides clear targets for modern neuroscience tools, which have the potential to reveal the constitution of affective phenomenal consciousness within the brain. Our concurrent working assumption is that this type of consciousness provided some critical raw materials for the construction of cognitive forms of experience, in higher regions of the brain.

It is important to note that each of the instinctual circuits generates not only stereotyped behaviours but also diverse feeling states, such as expectant interest, orgasmic delight, trepidatious fear, destructive rage, loving affection, sorrowful grief, and exuberant joy. Again, the critical evidence for this comes from the fact that these emotional states can be aroused by artificial electrical and chemical stimulation of the specific structures along these circuits, and they serve as specific rewards and punishments in the control of simple approach and withdrawal behaviours. The circuits for these basic emotions are conserved across the mammalian series, and they admit of considerable chemical specificity. It is important to note that these instinctual motivations are genetically built into the cross-mammalian foundations of the brain (Damasion, 1999b; Panksepp, 1998a). They are no less innate than the vital evolutionary survival and sexual needs that gave rise to them. They are unconditioned "tools for living". The emotional learning associated with these instincts is secondary to the instincts themselves (see Figure 10.1), permitting us to envision novel "Laws of Affect" that control learning.

To be clear, subcortical affective processes come in at least three major categorical forms: (a) the homeostatic internal bodily drives (such as hunger and thermoregulation); (b) the sensory affects, which help regulate those drives (such as the affective aspects of taste and feelings of coldness and warmth); and (c) the instinctual-emotional networks of the brain, which embody the action tools that ambulant organisms need to satisfy their affective drives in the outside world (such as searching for food and warmth). These instinctual "survival tools" include foraging for resources (SEEKING), reproductive eroticism (LUST), protection of the body (FEAR and RAGE), maternal devotion (CARE), separation distress (PANIC/GRIEF), and vigorous positive engagement with conspecifics (PLAY). This evidence-based affective-neuroscience taxonomy (Panksepp, 1998a, 2011) uses a capitalized nomenclature to distinguish the identified primary instinctual-affective subcortical networks of the brain from the various colloquial blends of everyday cognitive awareness— namely, the tertiary processes of Figure 10.1. Our main goal in this chapter is to provide a more solid foundation of the primary-process emotional mind for the clinical, cognitive, and social neurosciences than currently exists.

5.   Exteroceptive ego; interoceptive id

Having reviewed the two ways in which the body is represented in the brain, it is easy to recognize in the data the two major mental systems that were described in the classical Freudian models reviewed before. The external body corresponds to the "ego"; the internal body is the "id" (see Figure 10.6).

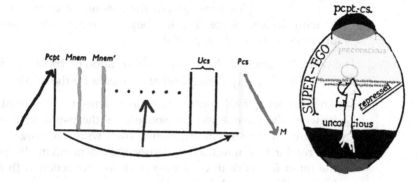

Figure 10.6. The preceding Figures 10.2 and 10.3 are coloured here to show some correspondences with the brain structures indicated by the same colours in Figures 10.4 and 10.5.

Freud himself said as much. About the bodily origin of the "ego" Freud wrote this:

> The ego is first and foremost a bodily ego; it is not merely a surface entity, but is itself the projection of a surface. If we wish to find an anatomical analogy for it we can best identify it with the "cortical homunculus" of the anatomists, which stands on its head in the cortex, sticks up its heels, faces backwards and, as we know, has its speech-area on the left-hand side. [Freud, 1923b, p. 26]

He elaborated:

> The ego is ultimately derived from bodily sensations, chiefly from those springing from the surface of the body. It may thus be regarded as a mental projection of the surface of the body, besides, as we have seen above [Figure 10.3], representing the superficies of the mental apparatus. [p. 26]

About the bodily origin of the "id", Freud wrote:

> The id, cut off from the external world, has a world of perception of its own. It detects with extraordinary acuteness certain changes in its interior, especially oscillations in the tension of its instinctual needs, and these changes become conscious as feelings in the pleasure–unpleasure series. It is hard to say, to be sure, by what means and with the help of what sensory terminal organs these perceptions come about. But it is an established fact that self-perceptions—coenesthetic feelings and feelings

of pleasure–unpleasure—govern the passage of events in the id with despotic force. The id obeys the inexorable pleasure principle. [1940a (1938), p. 198]

The word "instinctual" here is a mistranslation of *Triebe*. A *Trieb* is a "drive". Freud clearly defined what he meant by the term:

An "instinct" [*Trieb*] appears to us as a concept on the frontier between the mental and the somatic, as the psychical representative of the stimuli originating from within the organism and reaching the mind, as a measure of the demand made upon the mind for work in consequence of its connection with the body. [1915c, pp. 121–122]

It is evident that Freud himself readily "localized" the different bodily derivations of the ego and the id. We have only added anatomical detail (in Section 3) and clarified that there are within-brain needs, all of which distinctly arouse the body and, when aroused, continue to be modulated by the body. It is easy to recognize the functional equivalence between the brain mechanisms for exteroceptive representation and the bodily ego, on the one hand, and between those for interoceptive drive and the id, on the other. This applies equally to the interdependent hierarchical relationship between the two systems. These concepts therefore apply also to the brain processes that mediate bodily homeostasis and to those for the basic emotions, about which Freud said less. Still, Freud did envision the foundations of basic emotion in ways that reflect modern views:

And what is an affect in the dynamic sense? It is in any case something highly composite. An affect includes in the first place particular motor innervations or discharges and secondly certain feelings; the latter are of two kinds—perceptions of the motor actions that have occurred and the direct feelings of pleasure and unpleasure which, as we say, give the affect its keynote. But I do not think that with this enumeration we have arrived at the essence of an affect. We seem to see deeper in the case of some affects and to recognize that the core which holds the combination we have described together is the repetition of some particular significant experience. This experience could only be a very early impression of a very general nature, placed in the prehistory not of the individual but of the species. [1916–17, p. 395]

6.   The exteroceptive fallacy

The close parallelism between the brain mechanisms for the external and internal aspects of body representation, on the one hand, and the functional properties of the ego and id on the other, reveal a stark contradiction between current affective-neuroscience concepts of mind and those of Freud. In this respect Freud inaugurated the conflation of unconscious processes with cognitive unawareness of instinctual consciousness, thereby prematurely relegating unmonitored affective processes into the "unconscious" category (see Berlin, 2011, and the accompanying commentaries). As we will see, this practice oversimplifies the varieties of conscious and unconscious processes that actually exist.

To begin to expose this problem, we need to point out that Freud never questioned the classical assumption that consciousness was a cortical function:

> What consciousness yields consists essentially of perceptions of excitations coming from the external world and of feelings of pleasure and unpleasure which can only arise from within the mental apparatus; it is therefore possible to assign to the system *Pcpt.-Cs.* a position in space. It must lie on the borderline between inside and outside; it must be turned towards the external world and must envelop the other psychical systems. It will be seen that there is nothing daringly new in these assumptions; we have merely adopted the views on localization held by cerebral anatomy, which locates the "seat" of consciousness in the cerebral cortex—the outermost, enveloping layer of the central organ. Cerebral anatomy has no need to consider why, speaking anatomically, consciousness should be lodged on the surface of the brain instead of being safely housed somewhere in its inmost interior. [1920g, p. 24]

Freud recognized that consciousness also entailed an interoceptive, affective aspect. He even suggested that this aspect defined the original biological "purpose" of consciousness (1911b, p. 220). That is why Antonio Damasio was moved to say that "Freud's insights on the nature of affect are consonant with the most advanced contemporary neuroscience views" (Damasio, 1999a, p. 38).

But it is clear from the above quotation that even the affective aspect of consciousness was, for Freud, "lodged on the surface of the brain". Here he states this view even more explicitly:

> The process of something becoming conscious is above all linked with the perceptions which our sense organs receive from the external world. From the topographical point of view, therefore, it is a phenomenon which takes place in the outermost cortex of the ego. It is true that we also receive information from the inside of the body—the feelings, which actually exercise a more peremptory influence on our mental life than external perceptions; moreover, in certain circumstances the sense organs themselves transmit feelings, sensations of pain, in addition to the perceptions specific to them. Since, however, these sensations (as we call them in contrast to conscious perceptions) also emanate from the terminal organs and since we regard all these as prolongations or offshoots of the cortical layer, we are still able to maintain the assertion made above. The only distinction would be that, as regards the terminal organs of sensation and feeling, the body itself would take the place of the external world. [1940a (1938), pp. 161–162]

In making this assumption Freud followed a long tradition, which continues to this day. Consider for example the following remark made by Joseph LeDoux:

> When electrical stimuli applied to the amygdala of humans elicit feelings of fear . . ., it is not because the amygdala "feels" fear, but instead because the various networks that the amygdala activates ultimately provide working memory with inputs that are labeled as fear. This is all compatible with the Freudian notion that conscious emotion is the awareness of something that is basically unconscious. [1999, p. 46]

The latest incarnation of this "corticocentric" tradition is the work of Bud Craig (2009). He believes there is a cortical projection zone for the internal body, in the posterior insula, which he describes as the basis of the body-as-subject, the "self" (precisely the function we have attributed above, on the basis of a different research tradition, to the upper brainstem). We present this critique from the perspective that the locus of subjectivity does not reside in the insula, while conceding that many sensory affects (e.g., disgust)—

as opposed to primary-process basic emotions (Panksepp, 1998a, 2007, 2011)—and probably various other bodily sensations, along with certain sensory affects, are indeed processed by the insula (Panksepp, 2007).

7. Consciousness without cortex

Recent research demonstrates unequivocally that the corticocentric view of consciousness (and the subjective "self") is mistaken. Consider the following interview, reported at our Berlin congress by Damasio (2011a), concerning a patient in whom the insula was bilaterally (totally) obliterated by herpes simplex encephalitis. According to Craig's (2009) view, this patient should lack subjective, affective selfhood; he should lack the very page upon which experience is written. But this was not the case:

Q: "Do you have a sense of self?"

A: "Yes, I do."

Q: "What if I told you that you weren't here right now?"

A: "I'd say you've gone blind and deaf."

Q: "Do you think that other people can control your thoughts?"

A: "No."

Q: "And why do you think that's not possible?"

A: "You control your own mind, hopefully."

Q: "What if I were to tell you that your mind was the mind of somebody else?"

A: "When was the transplant, I mean, the brain transplant?"

Q: "What if I were to tell you that I know you better than you know yourself?"

A: "I would think you're wrong."

Q: "What if I were to tell you that you are aware that I'm aware?"

A: "I would say you're right."

Q: "You are aware that I am aware?"

A: "I am aware that you are aware that I am aware."

This case disproves only Craig's restricted (insular) version of the corticocentric theory. What about the rest of the cortex? In pre-clinical animal models, the removal of the neocortex has long been known to spare emotionality. Indeed, not only are the rewarding effects of subcortical brain stimulations demonstrably preserved in decorticated creatures, these animals are actually more emotional than normal (Huston & Borbely, 1973, 1974). The most strikingly concordant human evidence to emerge in recent years, relevant to this broader question, concerns a condition called hydranen-cephaly, in which the cerebral cortex as a whole is destroyed *in utero* (usually due to infarction in the entire territory of the anterior cerebral circulation) (Shewmon, Holmse, & Byrne, 1999). Autopsy studies reveal that islands of cortex that may be preserved in such cases (see Figure 10.7) are functionally disconnected from the thala-mus due to destruction of the linking white matter. The surviving cortical fragments are also gliotic and are therefore completely non-functional. This is confirmed by the clinical observation that, although visual cortex is preserved, the patients are blind (Merker,

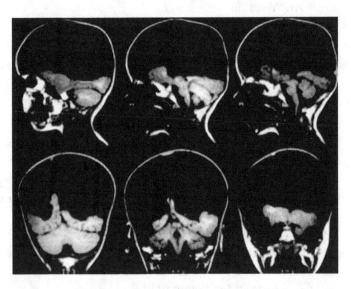

FIGURE 10.7.   A typical hydranencephalic brain. (Reprinted with permission of the American College of Radiology (ACR, 2004). No other representation of this material is authorized without expressed, written permission from the American College of Radiology.)

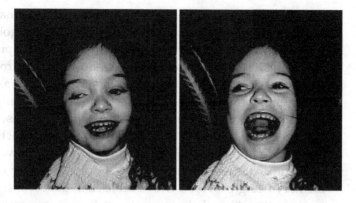

Figure 10.8. The emotional reaction of a young hydranencephalic girl. (We thank Bjorn Merker for the use of these photographs, reproduced with permission of the child's mother; Merker, 2008.)

2007). However, the subcortical networks are functional; thus, the children are markedly emotionally functional human beings (see Figure 10.8).

> They express pleasure by smiling and laughter, and aversion by "fussing" arching of the back and crying (in many gradations), their faces being animated by these emotional states. A familiar adult can employ this responsiveness to build up play sequences predictably progressing from smiling, through giggling, to laughter and great excitement on the part of the child. [Merker, 2007, p. 79]

They also show basic emotional learning. They:

> take behavioral initiatives within the severe limitations of their motor disabilities, in the form of instrumental behaviors such as making noise by kicking trinkets hanging in a special frame constructed for the purpose ("little room"), or activating favorite toys by switches, presumably based upon associative learning of the connection between actions and their effects. Such behaviors are accompanied by situationally appropriate signs of pleasure and excitement on the part of the child. [p. 79].

Although there is in these children significant degradation of the types of consciousness that are normally associated with external perception, there can be no doubt that they are conscious, both quantitatively and qualitatively. They are not only awake and alert, but also experience and express a full range of instinctual emotions. The raw affective self is, in short, fully present. The gold standard for affects in animals is that learned "reward" and "punishment" effects can be evoked by stimulating brain areas that arouse intense emotional displays, as can be seen in such children, as well as in decorticated animals. The fact that cortex is essentially absent in these cases proves unequivocally that affective consciousness is both generated and felt subcortically. This contradicts the theoretical assumptions of LeDoux and Craig quoted above, and those of Freud. Affective consciousness is not dependent on working memory being provided with unconscious subcortical inputs that are only then "labelled" as emotions. It is an intrinsic function of lower regions of the brain.

And this does not apply only to affective consciousness.

8.   All consciousness is endogenous

The "state" of consciousness as a whole is generated in the upper brainstem. We have known this for many years. A mere decade after the death of Freud, Moruzzi and Magoun (1949) first demonstrated that global consciousness, in the sense measured by EEG activation, is generated not by exteroceptive stimuli but endogenously, in a part of the upper brainstem then called the "reticular activating system". This was quickly confirmed by Penfield and Jasper, who recognized in absence attacks (mentioned above) "a unique opportunity to study the neuronal substratum of consciousness" (Penfield & Jasper, 1954, p. 480). Their extensive studies led them to the conclusion that obliteration of consciousness could only be reliably evoked by restricted damage to such upper brainstem sites (which they termed the "centrencephalic system"). They were also impressed by the fact that removal of large expanses of cortex under local anaesthetic, even total hemispherectomy, had limited effects on consciousness. Cortical removal did not interrupt the presence of the conscious "self", of conscious being, it merely deprived the patient of "certain forms of information" (p. 65). Lesions in the region of the upper brainstem, by contrast, totally and rapidly destroyed consciousness, just as the absence seizures did. These observations demonstrated a point of fundamental importance: all consciousness ultimately derives from upper brainstem sources. Contrary to LeDoux and the other corticocentric theorists, all the cortical varieties of consciousness depend upon the integrity of these subcortical structures, not the other way round. This in not to deny that higher cortical regions add much to consciousness. Of course they do. But the evolutionary "roots" of consciousness are to be found elsewhere, and they are probably affective [Panksepp, 1998a, 2005a).

The classic observations that underpin this important conclusion have stood the test of time, with greater anatomical precision being added (for review see Nieuwenhuys, Voogd, & van Huijzen, 2008). Significantly, the PAG appears to be a nodal point in the "centrencephalic system". This underscores the single fact that has changed in modern conceptions of this system: the brainstem structures that generate conscious "state" are not only responsible for the degree but also for the core quality of subjective being. The primal conscious "state" of mammals is intrinsically affective. It is this realization that will revolutionize consciousness studies in future years (Mesulam, 2000; Panksepp, 1998a).

To put it bluntly: consciousness is generated in the id. The classical conception is turned on its head. The cortex was not the initial generator of consciousness, but this is not widely recognized in consciousness studies. As the late Paul Grobstein said: "Is 'reflective awareness' a 'luxury' on top of consciousness? Or might it be that without which there is no internal experience at all?" (in Merry2e, 2008). This is the classic problem in consciousness studies that still prevents many scholars from accepting the evidence-based conclusion that "reflective awareness" is not the *sine qua non* of subjective experience. Failure to accept the evidence still allows many to assume that we have no right to conclude that human infants and other animals that cannot speak have affective experiences. Of course, deep science does not indulge in concepts such as "proof" but only in the "weight of evidence"; with that as the cardinal rule for scientific reasoning, the evidence for affective experiences in all non-speaking mammals has been quite overwhelming for a while (Panksepp, 1998a, 2005a, 2011). Perhaps this line of reasoning will soon need to be extended to some invertebrates (Huber, Panksepp, Nathaniel, Alcaro, & Panksepp, 2011). In contrast, there is no evidence that living neocortex alone, without subcortical supports, can have any subjective experiences at all (Parvizi & Damasio, 2003; Watt & Pincus, 2004).

9. *Mental solids*

What, then, does cortex contribute to consciousness? It is clear from the facts just reviewed that the consciousness attached to core affective states is not really intrinsic to the cortex but, rather, derives from deep subcortical sources. Neocortex without a brainstem can never be conscious. Although neocortex surely adds much to refined perceptual awareness, initial perceptual processing appears to be unconscious in itself (cf. blindsight) or it may have qualities that we do not readily recognize at the level of cognitive consciousness. Exteroceptive sensory systems at the subcortical (e.g., tectal) level may have little more than an affective and bodily orientation feel to them. An appropriate formulation of the relationship between perception and consciousness (which is, as we now know, endogenous, subjective, and fundamentally interoceptive in an affective kind of way) might therefore be: "I feel like this about that" (where "this" is consciousness and "that" is perception). Consciousness is, to use Damasio's term, thereby *extended* onto exteroception. It is possible that perceptual and higher cognitive forms of consciousness emerged in the neocortex upon an evolutionary foundation of affective consciousness (Shewmon, Holmse, & Byrne, 1999; Vandekerckhove & Panksepp, 2009). In other words, *anoetic* phenomenal experiences may have emerged before *noetic* forms of consciousness in brain-mind evolution (Panksepp, 1998b).

Moreover, much of what we have traditionally thought to be unconditioned about exteroceptive consciousness is actually learned. This has been well demonstrated by the research of Mriganka Sur, which shows that total removal of "visual" cortex in foetal mice (*in utero*) does not impair their adult vision at all, and redirecting visual input from occipital cortex to auditory cortex in ferrets leads to reorganization of the latter tissue to support completely competent vision (for review, see Sur & Rubenstein, 2005). Clearly, from a corticocentric viewpoint, this either means that sensory perception is completely learned, or that perceptual functionality is completely controlled by subcortical structures, with subtle developmental extensions of affective experience perhaps being the foremost vehicle. In short, one of the great mistakes of modern cognitive neuroscience may be the assumption that cortical consciousness is built on intrinsic "hard-wired" cognitive computational principles. The resolution of conscious experiences in the neocortex may be largely learned developmental/epigenetic functions of the brain. For instance, the critical originating features of supposedly intrinsic cognition capacities, like the so-called "language instinct", are more likely to be deeply affective—perhaps based on social-emotional "urges to communicate" feelings (Panksepp, 2009).

The fundamental contribution of cortex to consciousness in this respect is stabilization (and refinement) of the objects of perception and generating thinking and ideas. This contribution derives from the unrivalled capacity of cortex for representational forms of memory (in all of its varieties, both short- and long-term). To put it metaphorically, cortex transforms the fleeting, fugitive, wave-like states of consciousness into mental solids. It generates objects. (Freud called them "object-presentations".) Such stable representations, once established, can be innervated both externally and internally, thereby generating objects not only for perception but also for cognition. To be clear, the computations and memories underlying these representational processes are unconscious in themselves; however, when consciousness is extended to them, it (consciousness) is transformed by them into something stable, something that can be thought, something in the nature of crystal-clear perceptions that are transformed into ideas in working memory.

When we say that conscious perception expresses the formula "I feel like this about that" we are knowingly invoking Freud's idea that the forebrain is a "sympathetic ganglion", in the sense that exteroceptive consciousness and learning reflect and serve interoceptive needs. Learning arises from associations between interoceptive drives and exteroceptive representations, guided by the feelings generated by the affective experiences aroused by those representations. This is why they become conscious; the embodied subject must evaluate them. (The associations are, to a large extent, determined by the unconditioned categories of basic affects, but the representations themselves are not.)

The stability of such representations then enables them to be used to guide subsequent conscious behaviour (it enables them to be "held in mind"). The prototype for this in Freud's conception was "wishing" (e.g., Berridge, 1996, calls it "wanting"), which was in the first instance regulated by the "pleasure principle" but energized by a pervasive urge to seek resources, from nuts to knowledge, so to speak. Instinctual affective bodily drives and emotions are initially objectless (cf. the "SEEKING" concept of Panksepp, 1998a, 2005a), but sympathetic associative learning rapidly leads to remembered objects of desire "coming to mind". In other words, wished-for (or feared, etc.) objects are rendered conscious by dint of their "incentive salience" (determined by their biological meaning to the subject as in the way SEEKING leads to interaction with the pleasure–unpleasure aspects of the environment, which is the ultimate basis of consciousness). In this way, if left to its own devices, the pleasure principle would produce what Freud termed hallucinatory wish-fulfilments (the prototype of "primary-process" cognition). Hence, the evolutionary and developmental pressure to constrain incentive salience in perception through prediction-error coding (the "reality principle"—a higher, tertiary-order brain-mind process, in our terminology; see Figure 10.4) places inhibitory constraints on action. Such error coding must, again, be regulated by the homeostatic (affective) function of consciousness, which determines the biological valence of perceptions. The resultant inhibition—which perforce occurs at the motor end of the apparatus, where delayed responses must be sequenced—requires tolerance of frustrated affects, but it secures more efficient drive satisfaction in the long run (Freud called this the "constancy principle".) This defines the essence of the executive function expressed in working memory, in the sense that we generally theorize it today (a sense that Freud would have called secondary-process thinking, which he also described as "virtual action").

Freud's secondary process, as we know from Section 3, involved "binding" of "free" drive energies. This created a reservoir of tonic mental energies, utilized for functions (like thinking) that Freud attributed to the "ego". Carhart-Harris and Friston (2010) recently equated this reservoir with the default-mode network. In fact, Friston's work is grounded in the same Helmholtzian conception that Freud's was. His model of the Bayesian brain (in terms of which prediction-error or "surprise", equated with "free energy", is minimized through the encoding of better models of the world leading to better predictions; Kiebel & Friston, 2011) is therefore, in principle, entirely consistent with the model outlined here.

It is important to note that in this model, prediction error (mediated by the sensory affect of surprise), which increases incentive salience (and therefore conscious "presence" of the self) in perception, is a "bad" thing, biologically speaking. The more veridical the brain's generative model of the world, the less surprise (the less salience, the less consciousness, the more automaticity) the better. Freud called this the "Nirvana principle". We shall return to it in Section 10.

Before we can do so, however, we must point out that secondary-process thinking entails an important additional feature that may also be attributed to cortex. The wished-for object-presentations that literally "come to mind" in primary-process (hallucinatory) thinking are, according to Freud, re-represented at a different level in bound, secondary-process thinking (which from an evolutionary brain perspective, we call tertiary process). He called this level of representation "word-presentation". The value of word-presentations for Freud was that—although they, like all cognitive representations, are originally derived from perception (in this case, hearing)—their symbolic nature enables them to represent abstract relations between the concrete objects of thought ("which is what specially characterizes thoughts, and cannot be given visual expression": Freud, 1923b, p. 21). This renders secondary-process thinking far more efficient than the primary process. It also renders it "declarative".

This is the contribution of cortex. Indeed, as far as we know, all cortical functional specializations are developmental/epigenetic. The columns of cortex are initially almost identical in neuronal architecture, and the famous differences in Brodmann's areas probably arise from use-dependent plasticity. Metaphorically, cortical columns resemble the monotonous random-access memory (RAM) chips of digital computers. Can intrinsic biological consciousness originate there? Can the subjective aspects of mind really be computed? There is no consistent body of credible data to support either of these guiding assumptions of modern cognitive science. The prevailing Computational Theory of Mind seems fundamentally flawed. It remains a torso in search of a sophisticated neurobiological Affective Theory of Mind. The neocortex—the supposed repository of consciousness—is intrinsically unconscious, notwithstanding its remarkable capacity to generate the detailed and refined "mental solids" that obscure all else from view.

10.   The reflexive ego

We said in Section 2 that external body representation is made of the same "stuff" as the representation of other objects. The external bodily "self" is represented as a thing—"my body"—and is inscribed on the page of consciousness (derived from the internal body-as-subject) in much the same way as other objects. It is, in short, an external, stabilized, detailed representation of the subject of consciousness. It is not the subject itself. It is important to recognize that this conception of the self is an illusion, albeit an everyday one. The external body is not the owner or locus of consciousness. It is not really the subjective self; it is an objective representation of the self.

The subject of consciousness identifies itself with this external bodily representation in much the same way as a child might project herself into the animated figures she controls in a computer game. The representations rapidly come to be treated as if they were the self, but in reality they are not.

Here is some experimental evidence for the counterintuitive relation between the self and its external body. Petkova and Ehrsson (2008) reported a series of "body-swap" experiments in which cameras mounted over the eyes of other people or mannequins, transmitting images from their viewpoint to goggles mounted over the eyes of experimental subjects, rapidly created the illusion in the experimental subjects that the other body or mannequin was their own body. This illusion was so compelling that it persisted even when the subjects (projected into the other bodies) shook hands with their own bodies. The existence of this illusion was demonstrated objectively by the fact that when the other (illusory own) body and one's own body were both threatened with a knife, the emotional reaction (measured by heart rate and galvanic skin response) was greater for the illusory body.

The well-known "rubber-hand illusion" demonstrates the same relation between the self and the external body, albeit less dramatically. So does the inverse "phantom-limb" phenomenon. The anatomical basis of such phenomena (which place Freud's theory of "narcissism" on a new empirical footing) may be equated with the well-known fMRI (functional magnetic resonance imaging) findings to the effect that the shape and size of somatosensory and motor cortical homunculi (the acknowledged locus of Freud's "bodily ego") can be readily manipulated and can even be extended to include inanimate tools.

The secondary nature of external bodily representation is further demonstrated by many well-known "mirror-neuron" phenomena. Gallese's group has recently shown, for example, that schizophrenic patients are unable to reliably differentiate between their own movements and those of others, on the basis that mirror-neuron activity (which generates cortical mirages of the own body moving when somebody else's movements are observed) is not controlled by frontal inhibition in these patients (Ebisch et al., 2012).

The above phenomena demonstrate, first, that the external body is not a subject but an object and, second, that it is perceived in the same register as other objects. Something has to be added to simple perception before one's own body is differentiated from others.

In this connection, the role of prefrontal cortex in reflexive consciousness (a.k.a. secondary consciousness, access consciousness, declarative awareness, etc.) is surely germane. So is the role of prefrontal cortex in verbal re-representation (Figures 10.5 and 10.6). This level of representation (a.k.a. higher order thought) enables the subject of consciousness to separate itself as an object from other objects. We envisage the process involving three levels of experience: (a) the subjective or phenomenal level of the *anoetic* self as affect, a.k.a. first-person perspective; (b) the perceptual or representational level of the *noetic* self as an object, no different from other objects, a.k.a. second-person perspective; (c) the conceptual or re-representational level of the *autonoetic* self in relation to other objects—that is, perceived from an external perspective—a.k.a. third-person perspective.

The self of everyday cognition is therefore largely an abstraction. That is why the self is so effortlessly able to think about itself in relation to objects, in such everyday situations as "I am currently experiencing my self looking at an object".

The unrecognized gap between the primary subjective self and the re-representational abstracted self causes much confusion. Witness the famous example of Benjamin Libet recording a delay of up to 400 milliseconds between the physiological appearance of premotor activation and the voluntary decision to move. This is typically interpreted to mean that free will is an illusion, when in fact it shows only that reflexive re-representation of the self initiating a movement occurs somewhat later than the core self actually initiating it. Such confusion is avoided if we use different terms to refer to the different levels of self-experience. We might, for example, call the re-represented (prefrontal) self of everyday cognition the "declarative" noetic self, and the primary affective (brainstem) state of being might be called the "core" anoetic affective self. The intermediate (posterior cortical) somatosensory-motor self might then be called the "bodily" self. With autonoetic consciousness, we can have vast varieties of idiographic selves (Vandekerckhove & Panksepp, 2009).

Our major conclusion may now be stated thus: the core self, synonymous with Freud's "id", is the font of all consciousness; the declarative self, synonymous with Freud's "ego", is unconscious in itself. However, because the ego stabilizes the core consciousness generated by the id, by transforming affects into object representations and, more particularly, verbal object re-representations, we ordinarily think of ourselves as being conscious in the latter sense. This obscures the fact that our conscious thinking (and exteroceptive perceiving, which thinking re-represents) is constantly accompanied by low-level affects (some kind of residual "free energy" from which cognitive consciousness was constructed during developmental psychogenesis). However, the underlying primary, affective form of consciousness is literally invisible, so we have to translate it into perceptual-verbal imagery before we can "declare" its existence.

The dumb id, in short, knows more than it can admit. Small

wonder, therefore, that it is so regularly overlooked in contemporary cognitive science. But the id, unlike the ego, is only dumb in the glossopharyngeal sense. It constitutes the primary stuff from which minds are made—and cognitive science ignores it at its peril. We may safely say, without fear of contradiction, that were it not for the constant presence of affective feeling, conscious perceiving and thinking would either not exist or would gradually decay. This is just as well, because a mind unmotivated (and unguided) by feelings would be a hapless zombie, incapable of managing the basic tasks of life.

11.   If the id is conscious . . .

The realization that Freud's id is intrinsically conscious has massive implications for psychoanalysis, biological psychiatry, and our understanding of the nature of mind. This turn of events could be profound, not least because when Freud famously proclaimed "where id was, there shall ego be" (1933 [1932], p. 80) as the therapeutic goal of his "talking cure", he assumed that the ego enlightened the id. It now appears more likely that the opposite happens; reflexive "talking" is apt to dampen and constrain core consciousness. How is this fact to be reconciled with the stated aim of psychoanalytic therapy—namely, the undoing of repressions? And what are the implications for other approaches to psychotherapy and psychiatry?

To just begin to answer this question, it seems reasonable to suggest that repression must involve withdrawal of declarative awareness (*autonoetic* experience) from cognition. This has the effect of reducing an "episodic" cognitive process to an "associative" one. The subject of repression still activates the representations in question (the repressed "object relationships"), but the associative links no longer attract reflexive awareness. We recall that this is the original purpose of ego development: the goal of all learning is automatized mental processes, increased predictability, and reduced uncertainty or "surprise". It is the biological salience of prediction errors—probably mentally mediated by a variety of feelings in addition to actual surprise—that requires the affective presence of the id (of the biological self). As soon as the ego has mastered a mental task, the relevant associative algorithm is automatized. This, then, could be the mechanism of repression: it consists in a premature withdrawal of reflexive awareness, in automatization of a mental-behavioural algorithm before it actually fits the bill. This would result in prediction error and, therefore, the ongoing risk of the repressed material reawakening affective salience. This lays the foundations for a "return of the repressed", the classical mechanism of neurosis.

The therapeutic task of psychoanalysis, then, would be to undo repressions (to allow the affective distress associated with the repressed situation to emerge) in order to enable the reflexive subject to properly master it, and generate episodic representations adequate to the task, so that it may then be legitimately automatized.

Psychosis, on this model, entails an almost opposite mechanism. Psychotic states appear to flow from protracted failure to automatize predictive models of the world, again presumably due to their original inadequacy for the task. This does not account for the whole mechanism of psychotic states, but positive psychotic symptoms at least (the omnipotent "attempts at self-cure", as Freud called them) entail excessive salience (Kapur, 2003). These patients live in a perpetual state of surprise, against which they defend themselves with delusional certainties (Corlett, Taylor, Wang, Fletcher, & Krystal, 2010). As with neurotic patients, the therapeutic task is therefore to help these patients develop more adequate solutions to the tasks of life, but in the case of psychosis we are confronted by a mind that actually knows "less than it feels it does", rather than knowing "more than it admits". The problem is the constant presence of the id—the constant requirement for the biological self to affectively evaluate the meaning of experience. The therapeutic aim "where id was there shall ego be" therefore seems more appropriate for psychosis than neurosis.

Since most readers are not psychoanalysts though, we will briefly apply our therapeutic suggestions to the current state of cognitive neuroscience. Considering its breath-taking neglect of the affective dimension of the mind, and thereby of core consciousness itself, the most reassuring observation we can make about contemporary cognitive neuroscience is that it is not suffering from a psychosis. Cognitive neuroscience is neurotic; it suffers from repressions rather than delusions; it "knows more than it admits" rather than "less than it feels". Many aspects of mind, such as affective states, have been prematurely placed into the unconscious, even though they are experienced but rarely acknowledged or measured (for a full discussion of issues, see Berlin, 2011, and accompanying commentaries). Our task is therefore to gently draw the attention of our cognitive colleagues to the constant prediction errors this gives rise to and to help them to tolerate the ensuing distress, so that a more realistic, affectively based, predictive model of the brain may emerge.

12.   The deepest insight

The irony of the foregoing historical-scientific review is that Freud might appear to have done a disservice to psychology by denying consciousness its pride of place. But this is not really the case.

First, when Freud was confronted in 1938 by the behaviourist juggernaut that was about to sweep aside his life's work, he remarked that consciousness was:

> . . . a fact without parallel, which defies all explanation or description. Nevertheless, if anyone speaks of consciousness we know immediately and from our most personal experience what is meant by it. One extreme line of thought, exemplified in the American doctrine of behaviorism, thinks it possible to construct a psychology which disregards this fundamental fact! [1940a (1938), p. 157]

In this spirit, we redirect attention here to the primacy of consciousness in mental life and in brain research. This in no way diminishes the importance of deeply unconscious learning processes of the brain, and so on, and the endless peppercorns of facts that have been generated by the "neuroscience revolution". But it questions the attractions of ruthless reductionism, currently so popular in biological psychiatry, where investigators try to jump from brain facts to the cacophony of psychopathologies codified in successive DSMs, without explicit interest in the intervening role of the experienced mind itself. Future progress in this field requires us to recognize the fundamentally affective infrastructure of the mind and its pivotal role in psychiatric disorders. We should be devoting at least as much effort to clarifying the neurodynamics of the primary affective processes in psychiatric disorders as we do to their mindless and seemingly endless neural and genetic correlates (Panksepp, 2006).

Second, we must recall that embedded within the many statements that Freud made to the effect that consciousness (by which he seemed mainly to mean declarative consciousness) was a cortical function, he always acknowledged the exceptional role of affect. For example:

> The question, "How does a thing become conscious?" would be more advantageously stated: "How does a thing become preconscious?" And the answer would be: "Through becoming connected with the word-presentations corresponding to it." These word-presentations are residues of memories; they were at one time perceptions, and like all mnemic residues they can become perceptions again. Before we concern ourselves further with their nature, it dawns upon us like a new discovery that only something that has once been a Cs. perception can become conscious, and that anything arising from within (apart from feelings) that seeks to become conscious must try to transform itself into external perceptions: this becomes possible by means of memory-traces. [1923b, p. 20]

In other words, although Freud thought that affects, too, were (interoceptive) cortical perceptions, he recognized that they were felt *directly*. He did not share the view that they first needed to be exteroceptively represented, or read-out, or "labelled" in working memory, to exist (which seems nowadays to be the most common viewpoint in the cognitive science of emotions). In fact, for Freud affects could not be represented in the same way that external objects were. This set them apart from all cognitive processes:

> It is surely of the essence of an emotion that we should be aware of it, *i.e.*, that it should become known to consciousness. Thus the possibility of the attribute of unconsciousness would be completely excluded as far as emotions, feelings and affects are concerned. [1915e, p. 177]

It is to be hoped that the neuroscientific facts reviewed here will help to make sense of this observation, which, to Freud's credit, he always acknowledged, notwithstanding the theoretical difficulties it must have caused him.

We will close with the observation that more essential to Freud's successive models of the mind than the locus and extent of consciousness was his fundamentally dynamic conception of it, coupled with the dimension of depth (or hierarchy) in the mind. This is why Freud repeatedly stated that the assumption of "two different states of cathected energy in mental life: one in which the energy is tonically 'bound' and the other in which it is freely mobile and presses towards discharge" (1915e, p. 188) was the deepest insight he had ever gained:

> In my opinion this distinction represents the deepest insight we have gained up to the present into the nature of nervous energy, and I do not see how we can avoid making it. [p. 188]

This dynamic distinction is not only preserved in our affective-neuroscience update of Freud's views—along with much else—it is actually enhanced. The link between affectivity on the one hand and Helmholtz's troublesome "free" energy on the other seems to provide a red thread through Freud's work, linking him backwards to Helmholtz and forwards (via Feynman) to Friston. Considering this and the many other vistas opening up with the rediscovery of the embodied, instinctual brain—which must of necessity be constrained by the cognitive brain and its predictive modelling—it is difficult to imagine how the neuroscience and psychology of the future can be anything but neuropsychodynamic. As the cognitive science of the late-twentieth century is complemented by the affective neuroscience of the present, we are breaking through to a truly mental neuroscience and finally understanding that the brain is not merely an information-processing device but also a sentient, intentional being. Our animal behaviours are not "just" behaviours; in their primal affective forms they embody ancient mental processes that we share, at the very least, with all other mammals.

13.   In conclusion

Our goal here was to re-establish a primary-process affective foundation of mind to the higher mental apparatus that is receiving the lion's share of attention in cognitive science and cognitive neuroscience, as well as consciousness and psychoanalytic studies. We chose to frame our argument in classical Freudian psychoanalytic theory since, during the twentieth century, perhaps he came closest to the vision we have shared. Although he, in the modern vein, situated consciousness on top of the brain, the weight of evidence now indicates that raw affects arise from the "basement" of the brain. Our argument has been largely restricted to the basement, and we recognize that when it is interfaced with unconscious secondary learning-memory and the resulting affectively energized cognitive thought processes, there will be vast additional complexities to be faced, along with the possibility of many mereological fallacies (part–whole confusions and conflations), as discussed superbly by Bennett and Hacker, in their exceptional 2003 book.

Of course, primal emotions unfold in relation to individual lives, but they are built into the brain as nomothetic endogenous behavioural and affective resources of the organisms. We have not sought to address how these ancestral powers of the mind percolate through the subsequent idiographic layers of brain-mind emergence. Freud attempted to do that, but future cognitive neuroscience and related neurophenomenological consciousness studies will need to flesh out those processes, with a full recognition that the bottom-up developmental-epigenetic emergence of minds needs to provide a solid foundation for the vast complexities of the automatized top-down regulations and effortful conscious mental controls that a mature (fully constructed) mental apparatus permits and promotes (Figure 10.1).

Notes

1. Freud's use of this term differs from ours in Figure 10.1. Since Freud's "primary processes" include both unconditioned (primary) as well as our secondary unconscious learning and memory processes, his "secondary" level of analysis is closer to our "tertiary" level of brain–mind complexity.

2. These arcane mechanisms are best relegated to a footnote. Here is Freud's most succinct formulation of them: "Cathectic innervations are sent out and withdrawn in rapid periodic impulses from within to the completely

pervious system *Pcpt.-Cs.* (φ). So long as that system is cathected in this manner, it receives perceptions (which are accompanied by consciousness) and passes the excitation on to the unconscious mnemic systems (ψ), but as soon as the cathexis is withdrawn, consciousness is extinguished. . . . It is as though the unconscious stretches out feelers. . . . This discontinuous method of functioning of the system lies at the bottom of the origin of the concept of time" (1925a [1924], p. 231).

3. Here the term "unconscious" is used in the dynamic sense.

CHAPTER ELEVEN

A neuropsychoanalytic approach to the hard problem of consciousness

Mark Solms

1.   Introduction

Iwelcome this opportunity to sketch my approach to the hard problem of consciousness. I call this approach neuropsycho-analytic. I could also call it metaneuropsychological. I will explain later what I mean by these terms.

2.   *Visual consciousness versus consciousness itself*

I believe that the approach to consciousness taken by the main-stream of cognitive neuroscientists has been hampered by an exces-sive focus on exteroceptive, objectified forms of consciousness, especially *visual* consciousness. That approach gave rise to the "hard problem" in the first place (Chalmers, 1995a, 1995b). I think

---

This chapter was first published as Solms, M. (2014), "A neuropsychoana-lytical approach to the hard problem of consciousness", in *Journal of Integrative Neuroscience*, *13* (2): 1–13.

we will find the going easier if we focus instead on consciousness *itself*.

My starting point is the distinction between the *subject* of consciousness and *objects* of consciousness. Visual consciousness, like all exteroception, pertains to objects. However, consciousness of objects cannot exist without consciousness itself—without a conscious subject. Objects of consciousness must always be perceived by a conscious subject. If the subject loses consciousness, the objects disappear. The converse does not apply. That is why I prefer to focus on the subject of consciousness; it is the nub of the matter. Even if no one can point to it, subjectivity exists; it is part of nature, and it is the common ground of all experience.

(I am not saying that things in the world do not exist in themselves, independently of consciousness. All the evidence points in the opposite direction. I am saying only that in the absence of consciousness in general—an experiencing subject—there can be no visual consciousness.)

3. Consciousness of objects versus the reality of things

This is a useful place to remind ourselves that things in themselves (as opposed to our perceptions of things) do not possess visual quality. Vision is a property of the subject (cf. Zeki, 1993). We tend to think of objects as if they consist ontologically in the forms by which they are presented to us visually. We think of our visual image of the world as if it were, in a word, *reality*.

That is because human perception is dominated by vision, which happens for good reason: vision (especially at the cortical level) generates "mental solids", which yield more stable renditions of things than do any of the other modalities of perception (Solms, 2013).

Nevertheless, we think of reality—of the material world—as if it were defined by the qualities bestowed by these modalities. With our exteroceptive senses, we experience "matter" as being characterized by (visual) solidity, (tactile) tangibility, etc. We might experience and think differently if we were bats (cf. Nagel, 1974).

We would likewise have a totally different conception of reality if we possessed, say, only a sense of hearing; then we would presumably think that reality consists essentially in something like sound waves.

The quality we bestow on things depends on our observational perspective. For example, when you observe lightening visually, you see a flash; when you observe it aurally, you hear a clap of thunder. What, then, does lightning itself consist in? It consists in neither of these perceptual objects; *in reality* it is a geo-electrical process that manifests differently in different sense modalities. The best description of the real state of affairs requires *abstraction* from the perceptual data—in this case, an abstraction called "electricity" (the flow of electrons from negatively to positively charged fields).

If we extend the boundaries of human sensory capacity through artificial aids (like electron microscopes), we find that matter appears quite differently from how it looks to the naked eye. When we probe it to its core, we are driven to descriptions that transcend the properties of perception. In the end, we are driven to abstractions like "quarks", "weak force", "strong force", and so forth, and the very materiality of matter (its solidity, tangibility) disappears. This is a significant fact for the hard problem of consciousness, and I will return to it later.

For now, I want to conclude that the material attributes of objects are not absolute, they are relative. They can be shown to vary in relation to the observing subject, just as Einstein showed that the properties of space and time vary in relation to the velocity of the observer. The perceived materiality of reality varies in relation to the magnitude and position of the observer. If you expand the magnitude of the object by means of an electron microscope (thereby reducing the magnitude of the subject, relatively speaking), matter seems to lose its solidity and tangibility. Likewise, if you change the position of the object relative to the sensory surfaces of the observer, it acquires different "material" qualities—for example, when you listen to an object rather than look at it, it becomes transitory.

Since perceptions of reality must be distinguished from reality itself, from the thing being perceived, I also want to conclude from what I have said that the distinction between real and mental does not coincide with the distinction between perception and idea. Perception of reality is part of the mental domain, no less than cognition is (remembering reality, imagining reality, etc.).[1] This much is obvious, but it is not the way we commonly think. Common sense can be misleading—even (perhaps especially) to scientists.

The mental, then, consists in both perception and cognition. But that is by no means all it consists in. I will return to this point in Section 8.

4. Conscious versus mental

Before I shift focus from perception and cognition—which pertain to objects of consciousness—and address the subject of consciousness, the nub of the problem, I must draw another basic distinction that was overlooked by the philosophers who laid the foundations of modern psychology. If the findings of recent cognitive science have taught us anything, they have taught us that it is necessary to distinguish between conscious and *unconscious* mental processes. Not all mental processes are conscious. This was, of course, Freud's great insight.

This has massive implications for psychology. That is one of the reasons why I call my approach neuropsychoanalytic. If mental processes are not defined by consciousness, then what distinguishes mental from non-mental processes? What is the defining property of the mental? Freud's teacher, Brentano (1874), suggested that it was intentionality—"aboutness". But all representations are about something, including purely mechanical ones like photographs (Strawson, 1994). Furthermore, the concept of aboutness is too bound up with the objects of consciousness. I think the mental is more intrinsically bound up with subjectivity.

The fact of unconscious mental processes applies equally to perception and cognition. It is possible to see without awareness[2] (blindsight), recognize without awareness, read without awareness, learn without awareness, remember without awareness, make decisions without awareness, and so on. In fact, just about every perceptual and cognitive task can be performed without awareness (Bargh, 2014).

Please note that such tasks pertain to the processing of representations. This implies that not only associative but also representational processing can operate unconsciously. Reading of words and recognizing of faces, for example, can readily occur with zero-prime subliminal presentation of the stimuli, where the subject is completely unaware of having perceived any stimulus at all (i.e., where there is no visual consciousness of the stimulus). But such tasks require detailed and precise representational mapping and symbolic decoding of the spatial configuration of the stimulus; in other words they require cortex. (I am unaware of any evidence for the notion that it is possible to read without cortex.)

These facts have two implications. First, they lead to the conclusion that higher cortical functions are not intrinsically conscious. Second, they beg the question: what is consciousness for? What does consciousness add to the already impressive capacities of unconscious perception and cognition?

5.   Higher cortical functions
are not intrinsically conscious

Actually, this has been known for a long time. Moruzzi and Magoun (1949) and Magoun (1952) found decades ago—apparently to their own surprise—that cortical activity in cats was driven not by external sensory stimulation but endogenously, from the brainstem below. The same applies to all other animals, including humans. Penfield and Jasper (1954), for example, concluded that human consciousness depends upon the integrity, not of cortex, but, rather, a part of the upper brainstem they called the "centrencephalic" region. The most striking recent evidence for this conclusion is provided by accounts of the behaviour of hydranencephalic children, born without cortex (Merker, 2007; Shewmon, Holmse & Byrne, 1999). These children (like all decorticated mammals) possess a normal sleep–waking cycle. They also show absence seizures, in which consciousness is lost and regained. They also display a full range of basic emotions, such as fear, joy, and anger. (In fact, decorticate creatures in general are *excessively* emotional; Bard, 1934.)

The main thing to notice is that the representational functions performed by cortex—the so-called "organ of the mind"—are *not intrinsically conscious*. I think the central function of cortex is not consciousness but, rather, memory—memory of a kind that enables detailed and precise and *stable* representations to be held in mind, whether they be conscious or not.

6. *The hard problem versus the easy problem*

Before turning to the question "what is consciousness for?" I want to address another issue that has just arisen. When I say that consciousness depends on the integrity, not of cortex, but, rather, of upper brainstem structures, I am locating the generation of consciousness in space (I am *correlating* mind with matter—the easy problem; Chalmers, 1995a, 1995b). I am also attributing the generating of consciousness to neuronal processes that occur in that space (matter *causing* mind—the hard problem; Chalmers, 1995a, 1995b).

I believe it is a mistake to do this, to say that neuronal processes "generate" consciousness. This mistake gives rise to the hard problem, which derives from our conflation of matter (solidity, tangibility, etc.) with reality, in the sense described above—caused by our privileging of exteroceptive ways of thinking. Because we privilege vision, we imagine that the object of the mind *as perceived visually* (i.e., the brain) causes or generates all the other modalities of consciousness, even consciousness itself.

In exteroception, everything depends on the relative position and magnitude of the observer—on the observational perspective of the subject. In the case of the mind–body problem, that observational perspective is reflexive. The subject is looking at itself in the (mainly visual) form of an external object. The subject of consciousness thereby represents itself as an object of consciousness. The body-as-subject represents itself as body-as-object.

Subjective consciousness arises from *being* the portion of reality that generates consciousness. The relationship between *seeing* that portion of reality—representing it visually as, say, the innervations of the centrencephalic region—and simultaneously *feeling*[3] it, is not a causal relationship. They are two manifestations of the same thing. It makes no sense to ask: how does an object of consciousness cause the subject of consciousness? (This is the hard problem.) That question (the hard problem) is even worse than asking: how does a flash of lightning cause a clap of thunder? I say "even worse" because the (visual) flash and (auditory) clap are at least *parallel forms* of consciousness—objects of consciousness—whereas the functional anatomy of the centrencephalic region is a visually perceived and remembered object *embedded within* the subjective being of consciousness—which is, if anything, a hierarchical relationship opposite to the one dictated by common sense. Consciousness causes (or enables) a conscious perceptual solid—not the other way round.

Be that as it may, consciousness (in all its manifestations) must in reality be generated by processes that lie beyond consciousness. We can only *infer* those processes from the data of consciousness.

In doing so, we would of course be well advised to make use of the data provided by *all* the modalities of consciousness, including what it feels like to *be* conscious. Moreover, we would be well advised to describe the processes underlying consciousness in terms that transcend the qualities of the sense modalities—that is, we should describe this portion of reality, like all others, in abstract terms. We should describe the reality of the mind (the lawful relations that we infer from the data of consciousness) in non-perceptual language, ultimately using terms like "energy", and so forth, as the physicists do. The reality described by physicists and biologists and psychologists is, after all, the same old reality, and the laws inferred via our different perspectives on it must eventually be reconcilable with each other. The mind is not made of different stuff from the rest of the universe. The only difference about the mind is that we have an additional perspective on it: because we *are* the mind, we know what it feels like to be a mind.

This is the essence of the neuropsychoanalytic approach. It makes use of both objective and subjective data of consciousness, and where necessary it prioritizes the subjective (the ground of experience). This is also why I use the term metaneuropsychology. A metaneuropsychological account of the mind goes beyond (meta) our material (neuro) and subjective (psychological) observations of it; it describes the real unconscious stuff of the mind in abstract terms, as a "mental apparatus"—following Freud (1900a).

I hope what I am saying is clear. It is not easy to set out the neuropsychoanalytic approach, because we are not used to thinking like this. Common sense dictates that reality is identical with what we see. Seeing is indeed believing, but it is not reality. Seeing takes place in the mind.[4]

7. So, what is consciousness for?

I will begin to answer the question from the exteroceptive (representational, mnemic) end of the mental apparatus, although I actually believe that consciousness is an endogenous property (and something fleeting and fugitive).

What consciousness bestows on the objects of perception and cognition is *attention*. Consider the phenomenon of "attentional blindness": if you do not attend to something in your visual field (even a person in a gorilla suit), it does not enter your consciousness. The same applies to cognition. Remembering, recognizing, judging, navigating, thinking, and so forth go on all the time, but these processes only becomes conscious when we pay attention to them. And we only pay attention to them when we *need* to. So the question, "what is consciousness for?" may be recast: why do we pay attention to some perceptual/cognitive processes but not others?

The answer is that we pay attention to the salient ones, to the ones that matter to us. What matters to us living creatures—we infer, following Darwin—are at bottom the things that affect our chances of surviving to reproduce. But this cannot mean that we pay attention to everything that matters to us. That would be impossible. We know empirically that consciousness is a very small place; we simply cannot "hold in [conscious] mind" everything we need to (Bargh & Chartrand 1999). The purpose of conscious exteroception, then, is to *master* the things that matter to us, in such a way that we *no longer* need to pay attention to them—in such a way that we may render them *unconscious* again. Conscious processing of object relations is a *temporary* state. (The ultimate aim of all cognition is zombiedom; Solms & Panksepp, 2012.) In other words, we seek through consciousness to establish predictive algorithms that render consciousness redundant. We seek to establish algorithms that work *automatically*: "when that happens, I do this". Freud (1911b) called this achievement the "reality principle": through learning from experience, we establish internal models of reality so as to be equipped to meet our needs there. Realistic solutions to life's problems only require the conscious presence of the subject when they fail, when things do not go according to plan.[5]

Salient things, then, are the things we did not, or cannot, predict—things that unsettle our equilibrium—the things that generate *uncertainty*. Friston (2010) calls such things "surprises".

There are roughly two types of surprise. Things go either better or worse than expected. The determining of this distinction, it appears, is what consciousness is for. Consciousness informs the subject, in real time, what to make of unexpected events (of their *meaning*). It enables the subject to feel its way through unknown quantities (deviations from homeostatic set-points) by answering the question: "is this good or bad for me?" The answer to the question—is this good or bad for my survival and reproductive success?—is provided by feelings: the things that are good for us feel "good" (pleasurable) and the things that are bad feel "bad" (unpleasurable).

It is no simple matter to calculate the biological meaning of unexpected events, as they happen, across the multiplicity of vital needs: nutritional, thermal, sexual, and so forth. This is what feelings provide. They provide an immediate global valuation of biological "state" (Mesulam, 2000). And they orientate the subject to what it should do in response to the unexpected events (e.g., approach versus withdraw). They provide a global assessment along the lines: "this is what the current situation means to me".

It is important to recognize that this assessment is determined interoceptively: "what does this mean *to me*?" This assessment of the state of the subject is then "extended" (Damasio, 2010) onto the data of perception and cognition: "I feel like this (good or bad) *about that*". This is what consciousness adds to exteroceptive perception and cognition. It adds subjective feeling and valence to representations.

Valence is intrinsically qualitative and, in this instance, intrinsically subjective too. That is why the objective properties of sensory stimuli and processes predict nothing about the associated qualia (cf. the qualia problem). The qualia belong to the subject. That is also why they feel as if they belong "to me" (cf. the binding problem).

The adaptive value of qualia is obvious. Feelings determine the subject's response to events that were not predicted by evolution (by "reflex" or "instinct") or by prior individual experience (by "conditioning"). Most events, of course, cannot be predicted by evolution and responded to automatically. Our enhanced capacity to deal with unpredictability (learning guided by feelings) is what distinguishes us humans from, say, ants.

8.   The anatomy of consciousness

It is no surprise, in light of what I have said, to find that the neural correlates of consciousness (the so-called generators of consciousness) *are located in the upper brainstem, in close proximity and in tight connection with the brainstem structures that monitor the state of the visceral body (i.e., the subject)—the state of the internal milieu, of our vital functions* (Damasio & Carvalho, 2013; Panksepp, 1998a). As Freud (1911b) surmised even earlier, the function of conscious feeling—of pleasure and unpleasure—is to detect oscillations in the tensions of our internal drive needs. The resultant feelings, in turn, have a compulsive influence on our actions. This is the "pleasure principle".

> The id, cut off from the external world, has a world of perception of its own. It detects with extraordinary acuteness certain changes in its interior, especially oscillations in the tension of its instinctual needs, and these changes become conscious as feelings in the pleasure–unpleasure series. It is hard to say, to be sure, by what means and with the help of what sensory terminal organs these perceptions come about. But it is an established fact that self-perceptions—coenaesthetic feelings and feelings of pleasure–unpleasure—govern the passage of events in the id with despotic force. The id obeys the inexorable pleasure principle. [Freud, 1940a (1938), p. 198]

When Moruzzi and Magoun (1949) originally identified the anatomical location of the brainstem generators of consciousness, they made the mistake of describing their function in purely quantitative terms, in terms of the *level* of consciousness, or "wakefulness". They assumed that the *contents* of consciousness attached only to cortical processes. It fell to more recent investigators (Damasio, 2010; Panksepp, 1998a) to recognize that *it feels like something to be awake*. These investigators recognized that the background state of consciousness—the subject of consciousness, *being* conscious—is intrinsically *affective*. Affective consciousness is secondarily extended upwards, to sample and test learned representations of the outside world, and thereby to determine the meaning of ongoing perceptions and cognitions (see Solms, 2013).

> Cathectic innervations are sent out and withdrawn in rapid periodic impulses from within into the completely pervious system [for perception]. So long as that system is cathected in this manner it receives perceptions (which are accompanied by consciousness) and passes the excitation onwards to the unconscious mnemic systems; but as soon as the cathexis is withdrawn, consciousness is extinguished and the functioning of the system comes to a standstill. It is as though the [id] stretches out feelers, through the medium of the system [for perception], towards the external world and hastily withdraws them as soon as they have sampled the excitations coming from it. [Freud 1925a (1924), p. 231; with acronyms spelled out in square brackets]

It is nothing short of astonishing that cognitive science overlooks the affective states that colour the whole of experience—provide the global background of all experience, the very page upon which exteroceptive consciousness is written.

It is important to recognize, though, that this background state of consciousness consists in more than the pleasure–unpleasure series, generated (in the sense clarified above, in Section 6) at the level of the upper brainstem. That simple form of consciousness—positive versus negative hedonic valence—appears to have evolved at least 525 million years ago, as its functional anatomy is shared by all vertebrates. It is not surprising that evolutionary pressures gave rise to more subtle affective distinctions; there are more than two meanings in the world (good vs. bad) demanding more than two types of response (approach vs. withdrawal). That is why we find, above the upper brainstem, a variety of instinctual-emotional circuits giving rise to a great many other affects and attendant actions. The general classes of affective circuits range from simple "homeostatic affects", like hunger and thirst, to the so-called "basic emotions", which Panksepp (1998a) capitalizes as SEEKING, FEAR, RAGE, and so forth. These latter circuits provide hard-wired psychological links between the inner and outer worlds. (We cannot afford—biologically speaking—to each of us learn from experience how to forage, flee, and attack.) The general classes of affective circuits also include what Panksepp calls the "sensory affects": pain, surprise, disgust, and so forth.

Added to all this, by dint of the precise and detailed representational capacities afforded by the vast memory space of cortex, is the extended consciousness of everyday perception and cognition—the mental solids of working memory, which threaten to hide everything else from view. (One is reminded of Plato's cave.) As I have said already, this form of consciousness (object consciousness) arises when consciousness itself (the subject of consciousness) samples representations of the external things affecting it: "I feel like this about that." Representations of the "thats" in question can be held in mind (in working *memory*) while we try to master the feelings associated with them (i.e., while we master their biological impact on us). Then, once we have mastered them—that is, when we have established a predictive algorithm that works, and automatized the adequate response pattern—we pay no further attention to them, and we render them unconscious once more. This important function—temporarily conscious perception/cognition—is not to be sneezed at, but, as already stated, it unfortunately tends to blind us as to the actually invisible, subjective, affective nature of consciousness itself.

The objects of consciousness are the stabilized mnemic imprints that meaningful sensory constellations make on our affects. However, since the purpose of such imprints (mental solids) is for us to learn how to meet our needs in reality, they are far from unimportant. That is why decorticate animals are excessively emotional.[6]

9.   The physiology of consciousness

The hard problem now boils down to trying to abstract the underlying processes that we experience as consciousness. We have two points of access to these processes: one provided (mainly) by vision and the other by affect. That is, we have "solid" images of the relevant neural processes, and we have feelings that correlate with them. The common denominator between these two terminal points of our knowledge appears to be *uncertainty*. This is the abstraction we are looking for.

In this connection, I would like to cite Freud's dictum: "consciousness arises instead of a memory-trace" (Freud, 1920g, p. 25). When you know what to do (have already learnt what to do), there is no need for affective presence, and therefore no need for consciousness. The memory trace does its job automatically.

It is only in the presence of surprise—in Friston's sense—that the memory trace (the perceptual/cognitive representation) must be brought back to awareness, through hyperactivation by upper brainstem mechanisms (especially midbrain, hypothalamus, and thalamus), and evaluated afresh. This amounts to a *temporary dissolution of the established long-term memory algorithm* (to consciousness arising instead of a memory trace). Physiologically speaking, this process coincides with the re-emergence of *lability* within the cells, and cellular networks (especially in basal ganglia—amygdala, nucleus accumbens, bed nuclei of the stria terminalis, septal nuclei—and hippocampus), until the revised trace is "reconsolidated" (Misanin, Miller, & Lewis, 1968; Tronson & Taylor, 2007).

There is, of course, a great deal more to be explained, especially with regard to the physiological details. However, it is important to remember that what we must discern behind these details is an abstraction. The requisite abstraction will explain all the observable facts, including our testable predictions. That is how science works.

10.   Hallucinatory wish-fulfilment

Since I am attempting here to sketch my neuropsychoanalytic approach only in broad outline, so as not to lose sight of the wood for the trees, I will limit myself—before closing—to the following further point.

Perception, according to Friston, Adams, Perrinet, and Breakspear (2012) following Helmholtz (1866), is an active process of hypothesis-testing, by means of which we seek to confirm our predictive models of the world. I have argued that *conscious* perception occurs when our predictions are *disconfirmed*, or in conditions where prediction is impossible—that is, in conditions of uncertainty.

I would like to add that this means we constantly SEEK (in Panksepp's sense) to confirm our predictions. SEEKING (which manifests largely as foraging in lower animals) is expressed largely as saccadic eye movements in humans (Panksepp & Biven, 2012). Saccadic scanning may be considered a visual form of foraging (just as whisker-twitching is a proxy for SEEKING in waking or sleeping rodents), a form of hypothesis testing.

The role of *dopamine* in such behaviour is well established. Of special interest, therefore, are the implications of this form of uncertainty—SEEKING to confirm predictions—for the mechanism of hallucination and delusion (for "wishful thinking"). The analogy with REM sleep and dreaming is obvious (Perogamvros & Schwartz, 2012).

Of incidental interest in this connection is the fact that completely immobilized eyeballs rapidly become blind; the photosensitive cells give rise to no new stimuli (to a completely predictable state of affairs, as far as the central organ is concerned).

11. Conclusion

Consciousness registers *the state of the subject* within biological scales of values. The primal form of consciousness is a phenomenon known generally as affect. Pleasurable affect means "biologically good" and unpleasure means "biologically bad". There are many sub-varieties of the biological good and bad with subtler meanings (e.g., panic means "beware: potential loss of an attachment figure").

Perceptual/cognitive representations are intrinsically unconscious sensorimotor algorithms (learned predictions as to how your biological needs can be met in the world). Consciousness samples such representations in order to bestow meaning on them. Object representations are stable sensorimotor configurations that may be *held in mind*; they stabilize and shape consciousness into mental solids. Once meanings are established, the resultant predictions are automatized and rendered unconscious once more.

Prediction errors attract attention to the salient representations. This occurs through the generation of what Friston (2010), following Helmholtz (1866) and Freud (1911b), calls "free energy": entropy, lability, and uncertainty. This may be *visualized* as a cellular process—perhaps as decomposition of protein kinase M-zeta (PKMz; Sacktor, 2008)—but it is *felt* as consciousness. Consciousness persists, then, until a revised predictive model is reconsolidated (until the free energy is "bound"). Consciousness of representations is *predictive work in progress*. And, as we know, much of reality is unpredictable most of the time.

Notes

1. A defining feature of Descartes' *res extensa*—namely extension or dimensionality – applies also to his *res cogitans*, to the extent that it consists in representations derived from the outer world (the "impressions" of Hume and Locke). This conclusion is supported by recent mental imagery research; perception and imagination utilize the same representational structures. That is why, for example, the time taken to mentally rotate three-dimensional designs of increasing complexity tallies with the time taken in reality (Shepard & Metzler, 1971). Object representations are measurable, at least in principle. I believe that Descartes drew the distinction between mind and matter wrongly; he misconstrued the mind–body problem.

2. "Awareness" is an ambiguous term, which is often interpreted as knowing one is experiencing, rather than experiencing itself. Experiencing itself consists in qualia, not reflections upon qualia.

3. In the sense of what it feels like to be that thing; the consciousness of being that thing.

4. Ironically, naïve materialism turns out to be a kind of crypto-idealism in which the mental nature of conscious perception is overlooked, and the qualities of matter-as-it-looks are conflated with those of reality itself.

5. Freudian repression consists in the *premature* automatization of such algorithms, before they meet the dictates of the reality principle. This leads to the constant threat of "surprise" (and therefore affect) and the return of the repressed (Solms, 2013).

6. In humans, there is the very important additional regulatory function of language—symbolic re-representation—the bedrock of Freud's "secondary process" (see Freud, 1911b).

Conclusions

I am very pleased to have published this selection of my writings in the Psychoanalytic Ideas series of the Institute of Psychoanalysis, not least for the reason that I look upon it as acknowledgement of the interest now attaching to neuropsychoanalysis—a radical departure from the mainstream of psychoanalysis that was not initially welcomed.

When I first became acquainted in the 1980s with neurological and neurosurgical patients, it was almost impossible not to be fascinated and moved by the strange and profound psychological abnormalities they were struggling with. This is not surprising; the brain is, after all, the organ of the mind. What was surprising, however, was how little interest my neurological and neuropsychological colleagues showed in the subjective aspects of these patients' disorders. They seemed interested only in the medical aspects—what clues did the mental symptoms provide for diagnosis of the underlying brain pathology?—or the cognitive aspects, in the abnormalities of memory, language, problem-solving and the like that these patients displayed. It was is if they saw the brain either as just another bodily organ or as an information-processing device—something like a computer. They did not seem interested in the brain as the source of our sentient humanity. For me, this was what was most obviously special about the brain: it had the almost miraculous capacity not only to regulate bodily functions and solve problems like a computer, but also to reflect on its own state of being, to feel feelings, to have desires, to fall in love—in short, to be a person.

For me, therefore, what was interesting about these patients was not only their neurological pathology and cognitive disorders, but the effects of their brain diseases on their conception of themselves, their self-esteem, their world-view, their sense of reality, their relationships, their dreams.

I wanted to spend as much time with them as possible, in a naturalistic setting, so that I could observe them and get to know them *as people*. I therefore made a request in 1986, which my colleagues at the time saw as an act of professional suicide: I asked to spend as much of my clinical time as possible in our Department of Neurosurgery's brain and spine rehabilitation unit. Nobody wanted to work there; it was considered a dumping ground and the dead-end of a scientific career. But what it allowed me to do was to work with the patients over weeks and months, rather than the usual days or even just hours in an acute-care ward or outpatient department, which is the usual stomping ground of behavioural neurologists and neuropsychologists. It also gave me the opportunity to see how these patients behaved with each other, how they related to the staff with whom they were living, how they related to their families and other loved ones during visiting times, and how these relationships developed over the process of mourning their losses, and through the many other emotional challenges they had to contend with. It also enabled me to see how they responded to trips home and to their first tentative sojourns into the new, strange, and frightening outside world.

Not to diminish the scale of the human tragedy that these patients were grappling with, I have to say that I felt like a kid in a toy shop. What rapidly became apparent was not only that these patients, of course, dealt with their challenges in ways that were quite unlike anything you would normally see, in the healthy population and in psychiatric practice alike, but also that the aberrations and novelties in their ways of dealing with the world—and with their inner worlds—varied in systematic relationship with the site of the damage to their brains. That is to say, it rapidly became apparent that damage to different parts of the brain gave rise to alterations in the life of the mind—the whole mind—that were to a large extent regular and predictable. What this meant, as we should have expected, of course, was that not only the brain's cognitive information-processing capacities but all of its mental functions, including the organization of emotion, motivation, and personality, are represented in the brain in a systematic and lawful fashion. I now became fascinated with the possibility of being able to map some of these lawful relationships, by studying the structure of the personality changes occurring in these patients and piecing together the organization of normal functions from the differential psychic aberrations that were produced by damage to the different parts of the brain. In order to do this, I needed an appropriate method of investigation and an appropriate conceptual language, which I could use as a starting point for my investigations.

This was my point of entry into psychoanalysis.

For all its faults, no other discipline has devoted as much serious effort to the business of developing a systematic method for observing and investigating the inner life of the mind, and a language for describing it.

Armed with nothing more than the Penguin paperback edition of Freud's works, therefore, and with absolutely no psychoanalytic training or supervision, I set about trying to conduct amateur investigations of the inner worlds of my neurological and neurosurgical patients. (It was a full three years later that I began my formal psychoanalytic training.) I also enlisted the support of my wife in this work and got her to agree to turn it into her doctoral research dissertation, while I simultaneously made a special study of the changes in these patients' dream-life for my own doctoral research. (The products of these two dissertations are described in Parts I and III of this book.)

We did this by taking these patients into psychotherapy, somehow intuiting that this was the best way to gain access to their private thoughts and concerns, and perhaps the only way to get them to truthfully share their heartfelt phantasies and fears.

I hardly need to add that these patients really needed and welcomed psychotherapeutic help, as indeed did their families. It is one of the most shocking consequences of mind–brain dualism that patients who suffer strokes and brain tumours (and the like) are not routinely offered the same degree of psychological care as psychiatric patients are. These patients are considered brain patients, not mental patients. But as I said, brain patients have after all suffered damage to the very organ of their minds. They have to contend with the most confusing and incomprehensible—literally unbelievable—alterations in their mental life. Some of them lose, for example, the capacity to ever lay down a new memory again, or the capacity to tell the difference between a memory and a phantasy, or between a dream and a real event (see chapter 4). They might equally lose the ability to sequence events in time, or to tell where the different parts of their bodies are in space, or to know where the left-hand side of the body and the world have gone to, or to find their way from their bed to the toilet and back again. Some of them also do not comprehend the language that everyone around them is speaking, and cannot understand why, or do not realize, that nobody can comprehend what they themselves are saying, or do not recognize that the face in the mirror is their own. Some of them also lose the ability to feel anxiety, or desire, or interest in the world; or conversely, they lose the ability to inhibit fears or phantasies, and accordingly they act out wild pregenital wishes at the drop of a hat, without understanding why everyone around them thinks there is something wrong with that. They also might deny their most obvious deficits and try, for example, to walk on a paralysed leg; or they will insist that the paralysed leg belongs to you and not to themselves; or they might believe that they have grown a new leg alongside the paralysed one; or they might claim that the paralysed leg is a little baby that they are temporarily looking after; and so on (see chapter 5). And as you sit and listen to these patients, and try to understand the world in the way they see it, and discern the changes in the structure and dynamics of the mind that must lie behind that, so you cannot help but gradually piece together how the mind—as we understand it in psychoanalysis—is represented in the tissues of the brain.

And what could be more fascinating than that? And what could be more important for the scientific future of psychoanalysis than to grasp this opportunity, to link everything we have learnt over the past 120 years of purely clinical investigations with the anatomy and physiology of the brain, as we understand them today, and thereby take the opportunity to benefit from the enormous technological advances that have occurred in brain science since Freud first enthusiastically predicted that "someday" such a linkage would be possible?

It was for me personally the most astonishing surprise to witness the resistance and reluctance to grasp these opportunities that was displayed initially by so many of my psychoanalytic colleagues. Fortunately, that resistance has gradually diminished, so that nowadays we have several groups of analysts working clinically with neurological patients, in different cities around the world, confirming and extending and correcting the initial observations that my wife and I first reported in our book *Clinical Studies in Neuropsychoanalysis* (Kaplan-Solms & Solms, 2000). We also have an annual neuropsychoanalytic congress in different cities around the world, regularly attended by hundreds of analysts.

As I have already said, alongside this clinico-anatomical research into the personality changes that occur with focal brain lesions, which I have always seen as the bedrock of neuropsychoanalysis, I also conducted clinico-anatomical research into the brain mechanisms of dreaming. I chose the function of dreaming for obvious reasons: because dream theory played such a fundamental part in the development of psychoanalytic theory as a whole, I reasoned that if we could understand how the brain generates dreams we could neurologically localize all the major building blocks of our model of the mind. I reasoned that this would also serve as a useful check on the reliability and validity of the inferences that I had made from our clinical investigations of the personality changes caused by focal brain lesions.

It was thrilling to learn that it was indeed possible to do this— that is, not only to understand how the brain generates dreams (while at the same time confirming the results of our other clinico-anatomical study), but also to realize that the broad brushstrokes of our basic psychoanalytic theory was consistent with this new research. That in turn led to important corrections in the prevailing neuroscientific view of dreams, which had the effect also of placing psychoanalytic theory firmly back on the scientific agenda. (In subsequent years, basic errors were also revealed in Freudian theory—see chapter 9—but that is how science works.)

It was sad to observe how much more ready my neuroscientific colleagues were to welcome psychoanalytic theories and methods back into the scientific fold, and to revise their thinking accordingly, than my psychoanalytic colleagues were to take on board the mountains of new and highly relevant evidence about how the mind works, emanating almost daily from neuroscientific laboratories around the world.

I hope that this book will go some way towards further correcting that embarrassing state of affairs.

In these closing remarks I have mentioned only two founding researchers in neuropsychoanalysis: myself and my wife. Many other people have since built on that work, and in the process they have greatly expanded the horizons of psychoanalysis, not only to encompass other topics but also other spheres of scientific influence. Their names appear repeatedly in the references cited in this volume, and a few of the publications were co-authored with them. My outstanding early collaborators were Oliver Turnbull, Katerina Fotopoulou, and Jaak Panksepp, but there have been many others in more recent years. I particularly want to recognize the voluntary work of the executive committee of the Neuropsychoanalysis Association (affectionately known as the Action Group) and its various international affiliates, such as the Neuropsychoanalysis Fund in London, the Neuropsychoanalysis Foundation in New York, and the Neuropsychoanalysis Trust in Cape Town. I also want to acknowledge the generous financial support that these organizations have received over the years from the Astor and Chapman families.

Above all else, the yield of our work in neuropsychoanalysis has been a significant shift in the field of neuropsychology as a whole, so much so that the very term "cognitive neuroscience" is becoming a misnomer for what we actually do. Some find it necessary nowadays to complement that term with a new term, denoting a sister discipline called "affective neuroscience", to take cognizance of the fact that we no longer treat the brain as if it were a mere computer (or a chemistry set, for that matter). The reality is that these two aspects of the mind are finally being melded into one, and the "big picture" concerning how the mind *really* works is coming into view. I hope that chapters 2, 9, and 10 give some sense of this.

We are living through a golden age in neuroscience, during a period of rapid breakthrough, in which we are finally recognizing and understanding that the brain is first and foremost a subject, not an object; that the most important features of the brain are its unique capacities for sentience, feeling, volition, free will, selfhood, and agency. These are properties that the brain shares with no other bodily organ, and indeed with no other object in the known universe. Surely, therefore, these are the features we should be concentrating on if we want to understand how this part of nature works. These features have been the subject matter of psychoanalysis for over 120 years now. Psychoanalysis therefore has a great deal to offer neuroscience at this point in its history, and that is why I decided 25 years ago to train as a psychoanalyst. I am delighted that such a large number of psychoanalytic colleagues are now recognizing this historic opportunity for what it is.

This is the moment that Freud was waiting for. As he once wrote to Albert Einstein, towards the end of his life: "It is not altogether a matter of regret that one has opted for psychology. There is no greater, richer, more mysterious matter, worthy of every effort of the human intellect, than the life of the mind."

REFERENCES

ACR (2004). *ACR Learning File: Neuroradiology* (2nd edition). Reston, VA: American College of Radiology.

Aglioti, S., Smania, N., Manfredi, M., & Berlucchi, G. (1996). Disownership of the left hand and objects related to it in a right brain damaged patient. *NeuroReport, 8*: 293–296.

Ainsworth, M. D. S., Blehar, M. C., Waters, E., & Wall, S. (1978). *Patterns of Attachment: A Psychological Study of the Strange Situation.* Hillsdale, NJ: Erlbaum.

Alcaro, A., Huber, R., & Panksepp, J. (2007). Behavioral functions of the mesolimbic dopaminergic system: An affective neuroethological perspective. *Brain Research Reviews, 56* (2): 283–321.

Antrobus, J. (1991). Dreaming: Cognitive processes during cortical activation and high afferent thresholds. *Psychological Review, 98*: 96–121.

APA (1994). *Diagnostic and Statistical Manual of Mental Disorders* (4th edition, Text revision). Washington, DC: American Psychiatric Association.

Aserinsky, E., & Kleitman, N. (1953). Regularly occurring periods of eye motility and concurrent phenomena during sleep. *Science, 118*: 273.

Aserinsky, E., & Kleitman, N. (1955), Two types of ocular motility during sleep. *Journal of Applied Physiology, 8*: 1.

Baler, R. D., & Volkow, N. D. (2006). Drug addiction: The neurobiology of disrupted self- control. *Trends in Molecular Medicine, 12* (12): 559–566.

Bard, P. (1934). On emotional expression after decortication with some remarks on certain theoretical views: Part 2. *Psychological Review, 41*: 424–449.

Bargh, J. (2014). Our unconscious mind. *Scientific American, 300*: 30–37.

Bargh, J., & Chartrand, T. (1999). The unbearable automaticity of being. *American Psychologist, 54*: 462–479.

Bazan, A. (2007). *Des fantômes dans la voix. Une hypothèse neuropsychanalytique sur la structure de l'inconscient voix psychanalytiques.* Montreal: Ed. Liber.

Bennett, M. R., & Hacker, P. M. S. (2003). *Philosophical Foundations of Neuroscience.* Malden, MA: Blackwell.

Bentall, R. (2003). *Madness Explained: Psychosis and Human Nature.* London: Penguin.

Bentall, R. (2009). *Doctoring the Mind.* London: Allen Lane.

Berger, H. (1929). Uber das Electrenkephalogramm des Menschen. *Archives fur Psychiatrie Nervenkrankheiten, 87*: 527–570.

Berlin, H. A. (2011). The neural basis of the dynamic unconscious [with commentaries]. *Neuropsychoanalysis, 13*: 5–31.

Bernroider, G., & Panksepp, J. (2011). Mirrors and feelings: Have you seen the actors outside? *Neuroscience & Biobehavioral Reviews, 35*: 2009–2016.

Bernstein, W. M. (2011). *A Basic Theory of Neuropsychoanalysis*. London: Karnac.

Berridge, K. C. (1996). Food reward: Brain substrates of wanting and liking. *Neuroscience & Biobehavioral Reviews, 20* (1): 1–25.

Berridge, K. C. (2007). The debate over dopamine's role in reward: The case for incentive salience. *Psychopharmacology, 191* (3): 391–431.

Berridge, K. C., & Robinson, T. E. (1998). What is the role of dopamine in reward: Hedonic impact, reward learning, or incentive salience? *Brain Research Reviews, 28* (3): 309–369.

Blass, R., & Carmeli, Z. (2007). The case against neuropsychoanalysis: On fallacies underlying psychoanalysis' latest scientific trend and its negative impact on psychoanalytic discourse. *International Journal of Psychoanalysis, 88* (Pt 1): 19–40.

Bodkin, J. A., Zornberg, G. L., Lukas, S. E., & Cole, J. O. (1995). Buprenorphine treatment of refractory depression. *Journal of Clinical Psychopharmacology, 15*: 49–57.

Bowlby, J. (1969). *Attachment and Loss, Vol. 1: Attachment*. London: Hogarth Press.

Bowlby, J. (1980). *Loss: Sadness and Depression*. New York: Basic Books.

Berger, M., Gray, J. A., & Roth, B. L. (2009). The expanded biology of serotonin. *Annual Review of Medicine, 60*: 355–366.

Bowman, C., & Turnbull, O. H. (2009). Schizotypy and flexible learning: A pre-requisite of creativity. *Philoctetes, 2*: 5–30.

Braun, A., Balkin, T. J., Wesensten, N. J., Carson, R. E., Varga, M., Baldwin, P., et al. (1997). Regional cerebral blood flow throughout the sleep–wake cycle. *Brain, 120*: 1173–1197.

Braun, A., Balkin, T. J., Wesensten, N. J., Gwadry, F., Carson, R. E., & Varga, M. (1998). Dissociated pattern of activity in visual cortices and their projections during human rapid eye movement sleep. *Science, 279*: 91.

Brentano, F. (1874). *Psychology from an Empirical Standpoint*, trans A. C. Rancurello, D. B. Terrell, & L. McAlister. London: Routledge, 1973.

British Psychoanalytical Society (2008). *English-Speaking Conference Debate*. London.

Cacioppo, J. T., Berntson, G. G., Sheridan, J. F., & McClintock, M. K. (2000). Multilevel integrative analyses of human behavior: Social neuroscience and the complementing nature of social and biological approaches. *Psychological Bulletin, 126*: 829–843.

Cacioppo, J. T., Penny, S., Visser, C., & Pickett, L. (Eds.) (2005). *Social Neuroscience: People Thinking about Thinking People*. Cambridge, MA: MIT Press.

Carhart-Harris, R., & Friston, K. (2010). The default-mode, ego-functions and free-energy: A neurobiological account of Freudian ideas. *Brain, 133*: 1265–1283.

Cavallero, C., Cicogna, P., Natale, V., Occhionero, M., & Zito, A. (1992). Slow wave sleep dreaming. *Sleep, 15*: 562–566.

Chalmers, D. J. (1995a). Facing up to the problem of consciousness. *Journal of Consciousness Studies, 2*: 200–219.

Chalmers, D. J. (1995b). The puzzle of conscious experience. *Scientific American, 273* (6): 80–86.

Chalmers, D. J. (1996). *The Conscious Mind: In Search of a Fundamental Theory*. New York: Oxford University Press.

Chen, J., Chen, P., & Chiang, Y. (2009). Molecular mechanism of psychostimulant addiction. *Chang Gung Medical Journal, 32* (2): 148–154.

Churchland, P. (1986). *Neurophilosophy: Toward a Unified Science of the Mind–Brain*. Cambridge, MA: MIT Press.

Coltheart, M., Curtis, B., Atkins, P., & Haller, M. (1993). Models of reading aloud: Dual-route and parallel-distributed-processing approaches. *Psychological Review, 100*: 589–608.

Corlett, P., Taylor, J., Wang, X.-J., Fletcher, P., & Krystal, J. (2010). Towards a neurobiology of delusions. *Progress in Neurobiology, 92*: 345–369.

Corrigall, J., & Wilkinson, H. (2003). *Revolutionary Connections: Psychotherapy and Neuroscience*. London: Karnac.

Cozolino, L. (2002). *The Neuroscience of Psychotherapy*. New York: W. W. Norton.

Craig, A. D. (2009). How do you feel—now? The anterior insula and human awareness. *Nature Reviews. Neuroscience, 10*: 59–70.

Damasio, A. R. (1994). *Descartes' Error: Emotion, Reason, and the Human Brain*. New York: Putnam's Sons.

Damasio, A. R. (1999a). Commentary [on J. Panksepp, "Emotions as viewed by psychoanalysis and neuroscience: An exercise in consilience"]. *Neuropsychoanalysis, 1*, 38–39.

Damasio, A. R. (1999b). *The Feeling of What Happens: Body and Emotion in the Making of Consciousness*. New York: Harcourt Brace.

Damasio, A. R. (2004). *Looking for Spinoza*. London: Vintage.

Damasio, A. R. (2010). *Self Comes to Mind*. New York: Pantheon.

Damasio, A. R. (2011a). *Constructing Selves*. Paper presented at the 12th International Neuropsychoanalysis Congress, Berlin, 23–26 June.

Damasio, A. R. (2011b). *Self Comes to Mind: Constructing the Conscious Brain*. London: Heinemann.

Damasio, A. R., & Carvalho, G. (2013). The nature of feelings: Evolutionary and neurobiological origins. *Nature Reviews. Neuroscience, 14*: 143–152.

Dawkins, R. (1998). *Unweaving the Rainbow*. London: Penguin.

Decety, J., & Cacioppo, J. T. (2011). *Handbook of Social Neuroscience*. New York: Oxford University Press.

De Kloet, E., Joels, M., & Holsboer, F. (2005). Stress and the brain: From adaptation to disease. *Nature Reviews. Neuroscience, 6*: 463–475.

Delgado, P. L., Charney, D. S., Price, L. H., Aghajanian, G. K., Landis, H., & Heninger, G. R. (1990). Serotonin function and the mechanism of antidepressant action: Reversal of antidepressant-induced remission by rapid depletion of plasma tryptophan. *Archives of General Psychiatry, 47*: 411–418.

Dement, W., & Kleitman, N. (1957a). Cyclic variations in EEG during sleep and their relation to eye movements, body mobility and dreaming. *Electroencephalography and Clinical Neurophysiology, 9*: 673.

Dement, W., & Kleitman, N. (1957b). The relation of eye movements during sleep to dream activity: An objective method for the study of dreaming. *Journal of Experimental Psychology, 53*: 89.

Dietrich, D., Fodor, G., Kastner, W., & Ulieru, M. (2007). *Considering a Technical Realization of a Neuro-Psychoanalytical Model of the Mind*. Conference Proceedings, 1st International Engineering and Neuro-Psychoanalysis Forum, Vienna, July.

Doidge, N. (2008). *The Brain That Changes Itself*. New York: Penguin.

Ebisch, S., Salone, A., Ferri, F., de Berardis, D., Romani, G. L., Ferro, F., et al. (2012). Out of touch with reality? Social perception in first-episode schizophrenia. *Social Cognitive and Affective Neuroscience, 7*. doi:10.1093/scan/nss012

Fechner, G. (1889). *Elemente der Psychophysik*. Leipzig: Breitkopf & Härtel.

Feinberg, T. (2001). *Altered Egos: How the Brain Creates the Self*. Oxford: Oxford University Press.

Feinberg, T., De Luca, J., Giacino, J., Roane, D., & Solms, M. (2005). Right hemisphere pathology and the self: Delusional misidentification and reduplication. In: T. Feinberg & J. Keenan (Eds.), *The Lost Self: Pathologies of the Brain and Identity* (pp. 100–130). New York: Oxford Universities Press.

Feldman, M. (1971). Physiological observations in a chronic case of "locked-in" syndrome. *Neurology, 21*: 459.

Ferris, C. F., Kulkarni, P., Sullivan, J. M., Jr., Harder, J. A., Messenger, T. L., & Febo, M. (2005). Pup suckling is more rewarding than cocaine: Evidence from functional magnetic resonance imaging and three-dimensional computational analysis. *Journal of Neuroscience, 25* (1): 149–156.

Finger, S. (1994). *Origins of Neuroscience: A History of Explorations into Brain Function*. New York: Oxford University Press.

Fonagy, P., Steele, H., & Steele, M. (1991). Maternal representations of attachment during pregnancy predict the organization of infant–mother attachment at one year of age. *Child Development, 62*: 891–905.

Fonagy, P., & Target, M. (1996). Playing with reality: I. Theory of mind and the normal development of psychic reality. *International Journal of Psychoanalysis, 77*: 217–233.

Fotopoulou, A. (2012). Towards psychodynamic neuroscience. In: A. Fotopoulou, M. Conway, & D. Pfaff (Eds.), *From the Couch to the Lab: Trends in Psychodynamic Neuroscience* (pp. 1–12). Oxford: Oxford University Press.

Fotopoulou, A., Conway, M. A., & Solms, M. (2007). Confabulation: Motivated reality monitoring. *Neuropsychologia, 45*: 2180–2190.

Fotopoulou, A., Conway, M. A., Solms, M., Tyrer, S., & Kopelman, M. (2008). Self-serving confabulation in prose recall. *Neuropsychologia, 46*: 1429–1441.

Fotopoulou, A., Conway, M. A., Tyrer, S., Birchall, D., Griffiths, P., & Solms, M. (2008). Is the content of confabulation positive? An experimental study. *Cortex, 44*: 764–772.

Fotopoulou, A., Pfaff, D., & Conway, M. A. (2012). *From the Couch to the Lab: Trends in Neuropsychoanalysis.* Oxford: Oxford University Press.

Fotopolou, A., Solms, M., & Turnbull, O. H. (2004). Wishful reality distortions in confabulation. *Neuropsychologia, 42*: 727–744.

Foulkes, D. (1962). Dream reports from different stages of sleep. *Journal of Abnormal and Social Psychology, 65*: 14.

Foulkes, D., Spear, P., & Symonds, J. (1966). Individual differences in mental activity at sleep onset. *Journal of Abnormal and Social Psychology., 71*: 280.

Foulkes, D., & Vogel, G. (1965). Mental activity at sleep onset. *Journal of Abnormal and Social Psychology, 70*: 231.

Frank, J. (1946). Clinical survey and results of 200 cases of prefrontal leucotomy. *Journal of Mental Science, 92*: 497.

Frank, J. (1950). Some aspects of lobotomy (prefrontal leucotomy) under psychoanalytic scrutiny. *Psychiatry: Interpersonal and Biological Processes, 13*: 35.

Freed, P. J., Yanagihara, T. K., Hirsch, J., & Mann, J. J. (2009). Neural mechanisms of grief regulation. *Biological Psychiatry, 66* (1): 33–40.

Freud, S. (1891). *On Aphasia: A Critical Study.* London: Imago, 1953.

Freud, S. (1894a). The neuro-psychoses of defence. *Standard Edition, 3*: 45–61.

Freud, S. (1895d) (with Breuer, J.). *Studies on Hysteria. Standard Edition, 2.*

Freud, S. (1898a). Sexuality in the aetiology of the neuroses. *Standard Edition, 3*: 261–286.

Freud, S. (1900a). *The Interpretation of Dreams. Standard Edition, 4/5.*

Freud, S. (1911b). Formulations on the two principles of mental functioning. *Standard Edition, 12*: 215–226.

Freud, S. (1914c). On narcissism: An introduction. *Standard Edition, 14.*

Freud, S. (1915c). *Instincts and Their Vicissitudes. Standard Edition, 14*: 117–140.

Freud, S. (1915e). The Unconscious. *Standard Edition, 14*: 166–204.

Freud, S. (1916–17). *Introductory Lectures on Psychoanalysis. Standard Edition, 15/16.*

Freud, S. (1917d [1915]). A metapsychological supplement to the theory of dreams. *Standard Edition, 14*: 222–235.

Freud, S. (1917e [1915]). Mourning and melancholia. *Standard Edition, 14*: 239–258.

Freud, S. (1920g). *Beyond the Pleasure Principle. Standard Edition, 18*: 7–64.

Freud, S. (1923a [1922]). Two encyclopaedia articles. *Standard Edition, 18*.

Freud, S. (1923b). *The Ego and the Id. Standard Edition, 19*: 12–59.

Freud, S. (1925a [1924]). A note on the "mystic writing pad". *Standard Edition, 16*: 227–232.

Freud, S. (1929). Letter to Einstein. In: I. Grubrich-Simitis, "No greater, richer, more mysterious subject [. . .] than the life of the mind": An early exchange of letters between Freud and Einstein. *International Journal of Psychoanalysis, 76* (1995): 115–122.

Freud, S. (1933 [1932]). *New Introductory Lectures on Psycho-Analysis. Standard Edition, 22*: 5–182.

Freud, S. (1940a [1938]). *An Outline of Psycho-Analysis. Standard Edition, 23*: 144–207.

Freud, S. (1950 [1892–1899]). Extracts from the Fliess papers. *Standard Edition, 1*: 173–280.

Freud, S. (1950 [1895]). Project for a scientific psychology. *Standard Edition, 1*: 281–397.

Friston, K. (2010). The free-energy principle: A unified brain theory? *Nature Reviews. Neuroscience, 11*: 127–138.

Friston, K., Adams, R., Perrinet, L., & Breakspear, M. (2012). Perceptions as hypotheses: Saccades as experiments. *Frontiers in Psychology, 3*: 151.

Gallese, V., Keysers, C., & Rizzolatti, G. (2004). A unifying view of the basis of social cognition. *Trends in Cognitive Science, 8*: 396–403.

Guterl, F. (2002). What Freud got right. *Newsweek*, November 5.

Haber, S. N., & Knutson, B. (2010). The reward circuit: Linking primate anatomy and human imaging. *Neuropsychopharmacology Reviews, 35* (1): 4–26.

Harlow, H. (1958). The nature of love. *American Psychologist, 13*: 673–685.

Harris, J. C. (1989). Experimental animal modeling of depression and anxiety. *Psychiatric Clinics of North America, 18*: 815–836.

Harro, J., & Oreland, L. (2001). Depression as a spreading adjustment disorder of monoaminergic neurons: A case for primary implications of the locus coeruleus, *Brain Research Reviews, 38*: 79–128.

Hartmann, B., Russ, D., Oldfield, M., Falke, R., & Skoff, B. (1980). Dream content: Effects of L-DOPA. *Sleep Research, 9*: 153.

Heilman, K. M., & Valenstein, E. (1979). *Clinical Neuropsychology*. Oxford. Oxford University Press.

Heim, C., & Nemeroff, C. (1999). The impact of early adverse experiences on brain systems involved in the pathophysiology of anxiety and affective disorders. *Biological Psychiatry, 46*: 1509–1522.

Helmholtz, H. von (1866). Concerning the perceptions in general. In: *Treatise on Physiological Optics* (3rd edition), trans. J. Southall. New York: Dover.

Hobson, J. A. (1988). *The Dreaming Brain*. New York: Basic Books.

Hobson, J. A. (2000). The new neuropsychology of sleep: Implications for psychoanalysis. *Neuropsychoanalysis, 1* (2): 157–183.

Hobson, J. A., & McCarley, R. W. (1977). The brain as a dream-state generator. *American Journal of Psychiatry, 134*: 1335.

Hobson, J. A., McCarley, R. W., & Wyzinski, P. W. (1975). Sleep cycle oscillation: Reciprocal discharge by two brainstem neuronal groups. *Science, 189*: 55–58.

Hobson, J. A., Stickgold, R., & Pace-Schott, E. (1998). The neuropsychology of REM sleep dreaming. *NeuroReport, 9* (3): 1–14.

Holstege, G. R., & Saper, C. B. (2005). Special Issue: The anatomy of the soul. *Journal of Comparative Neurology, 493*: 1–176.

Huber, R., Panksepp, J. B., Nathaniel, T., Alcaro, A., & Panksepp, J. (2011). Drug-sensitive reward in crayfish: An invertebrate model system for the study of SEEKING, reward, addiction, and withdrawal. *Neuroscience & Biobehavioral Reviews, 35*: 1847–1853.

Huston, J. P., & Borbely, A. A. (1973). Operant conditioning in forebrain ablated rats by use of rewarding hypothalamic stimulation. *Brain Research, 50*: 467–472.

Huston, J. P., & Borbely, A. A. (1974). The thalamic rat: General behavior, operant learning with rewarding hypothalamic stimulation, and effects of amphetamine. *Physiology & Behaviour, 12*: 433–448.

Janz, D. (1974). Epilepsy and the sleep–waking cycle. In: *Handbook of Clinical Neurology, Vol. 15*, ed. P. Vinken & G. Bruyn. Amsterdam: Elsevier.

Jones, B. (1979). Elimination of paradoxical sleep by lesions of the pontine gigantocellular tegmental field in the cat. *Neuroscience Letters, 13*: 285.

Jouvet, M. (1962). Recherches sur les structures nerveuses et les mécanismes responsables des differentes phases du sommeil physiologique. *Archives Italiennes de Biologie, 153*: 125.

Jus, A., Jus, K., Villeneuve, A., Pires, A., Lachance, R., Fortier, J., et al. (1973). Studies on dream recall in chronic schizophrenic patients after prefrontal lobotomy. *Biological Psychiatry, 6*: 275.

Kahneman, D. (2003). A perspective on judgement and choice. *American Psychologist, 58*: 697–720.

Kandel, E. R. (1998). A new intellectual framework for psychiatry. *American Journal of Psychiatry, 155*: 457–469.

Kandel, E. R. (1999). Biology and the future of psychoanalysis: A new intellectual framework for psychiatry revisited. *American Journal of Psychiatry, 156*: 505–524.

Kaplan-Solms, K., & Solms, M. (2000). *Clinical Studies in Neuro-Psychoanalysis: Introduction to a Depth Neuropsychology*. New York: Other Press.

Kapur, S. (2003). Psychosis as a state of aberrant salience: A framework linking biology, phenomenology, and pharmacology in schizophrenia. *American Journal of Psychiatry, 160*: 13–23.

Karlsson, G. (2010). *Psychoanalysis in a New Light*. Cambridge: Cambridge University Press.

Kassel, J. D. (Ed.) (2010). *Substance Abuse and Emotion* (pp. 137–168). Washington, DC: American Psychological Association.

Kellaway, P., & Frost, J. (1983). Biorythmic modulation of epileptic events. In: *Recent Advances in Epilepsy, Vol. 1* (pp. 139–154), ed. T. Pedley & B. Meldrum. Edinburgh: Churchill Livingstone.

Kertesz, A. (1983). *Localisation in Neuropsychology*. New York: Academic Press.

Kiebel, S. J., & Friston, K. J. (2011). Free energy and dendritic self-organization. *Frontiers in Systems Neuroscience, 5* (80): 1–13.

Klawans, H., Moskowitz, C., Lupton, N., & Scharf, B. (1978). Induction of dreams by levodopa. *Harefuah, 95* (2): 57–59.

Kline, N. S. (1959). *Major Problems and Needs in Psychopharmacology Frontiers*. Boston, MA: Little Brown.

Kohut, H. (2009). *The Restoration of the Self*. Chicago: Chicago University Press.

Kolb, B., & Whishaw, I. P. (1990). *Fundamentals of Human Neuropsychology*. New York: Freeman.

Kondo, T., Antrobus, J., & Fein, C. (1989). Later REM activation and sleep mentation. *Sleep Research, 18*: 147.

Korsakoff, S. (1887). *Ob alkogol'nom paraliche.* [Disturbance of psychic activity in alcoholic paralysis and its relation to the disturbance of the psychic sphere in multiple neuritis of nonalcoholic origin.] *Vestnik Klin. Psychiat. Neurol., 4* (2): 1–102.

Korsakoff, S. (1889). *Über eine besondere Form psychiser Störung kombiniert mit multipler Neuritis.* [On a particular form of psychic disturbance combined with multiple neuritis.] *Medizinskoje Obozrenije, 31* (13).

Kosslyn, S. (1994). *Image and Brain*. Cambridge, MA: MIT Press.

Koziek, M., Middlemas, D., & Bylund, D. (2008). Brain-derived neurotrophic factor and its receptor tropomyosin-related kinase B in the mechnism of action of antidepressant therapies. *Pharmacology & Therapeutics, 117*: 30–51.

Laufer, M. E. (1982). Female masturbation in adolescence and the development of the relationship to the body. *International Journal of Psychoanalysis, 63*: 295–302.

LeDoux, J. (1996). *The Emotional Brain*. New York: Touchstone.

LeDoux, J. (1999). Psychoanalytic theory: Clues from the brain. *Neuropsychoanalysis, 1*: 44–49.

LeDoux, J. (2000). Emotion circuits in the brain. *Annual Review of Neuroscience, 23*: 155–184.

Levinson, D. F. (2006). The genetics of depression: A review. *Biological Psychiatry, 60* (2): 84–92.

Luck, S. (2005). *An Introduction to the Event-Related Potential Technique.* Cambridge, MA: MIT Press.

Luria, A. R. (1966). *Higher Cortical Function in Man.* New York: Basic Books.

Luria, A. R. (1973). *The Working Brain.* Harmondsworth: Penguin.

Magoun, H. (1952). An ascending reticular activating system in the brain stem. *Archives of Neurology & Psychiatry, 67*: 145–154.

Mancia, M. (2006). *Psychoanalysis and Neuroscience.* Milan: Springer.

Maquet, P., Péters, J., Aerts, J., Deliore, G., Degueldre, C., Luxen, A., et al. (1996). Functional neuroanatomy of human rapid-eye-movement sleep and dreaming. *Nature, 383*: 163–166.

Mayberg, H. S., Lozano, A. M., Voon, V., McNeely, H. E., Seminowicz, D., Hamani, C., et al. (2005). Deep brain stimulation for treatment-resistant depression. *Neuron, 45* (5): 651–660.

McCarley, R. W., & Hobson, J. A. (1975). Neuronal excitability modulation over the sleep cycle: A structural and mathematical model. *Science, 189*: 58–60.

McCarley, R. W., & Hobson, J. A. (1977). The neurobiological origins of psychoanalytic dream theory. *American Journal of Psychiatry, 134*: 1211–1221.

McEwen, B. S. (2000). The neurobiology of stress: From serendipity to clinical relevance. *Brain Research, 886*: 172–189.

McEwen, B. S. (2007). Physiology and neurobiology of stress and adaptation: Central role of the brain. *Physiological Reviews, 87*: 873–904.

Merker, B. (2007). Consciousness without a cerebral cortex: A challenge for neuroscience and medicine. *Behavioral and Brain Sciences, 30*: 63–134.

Merker, B. (2008). Personal communication. Segeltorp, Sweden.

Merry2e (2008). *Conscious Children: A Brief Look at Hydranencephaly.* Available online at: http://serendip.brynmawr.edu/exchange/node/2355

Mesulam, M. M. (2000). Behavioral neuroanatomy: Large-scale networks, association cortex, frontal syndromes, the limbic system and hemispheric lateralization. In: *Principles of Behavioral and Cognitive Neurology* (2nd edition). New York: Oxford University Press.

Milner, A. D., & Goodale, M. A. (1993). Visual pathways to perception and action. *Progress in Brain Research, 95*: 317–337.

Misanin, J., Miller, R., & Lewis, D. (1968). Retrograde amnesia produced by electroconvulsive shock after reactivation of a consolidated memory trace. *Science, 160*: 554–558.

Morgane, P. J., & Panksepp, J. (1980). *Handbook of the Hypothalamus: Physiology of the Hypothalamus, Vol. 2.* New York: Marcel Dekker.

Moruzzi, G., & Magoun, H. (1949). Brain stem reticular formation and activation of the EEG. *Electroencephaloggraphy and Clinical Neurophysiology, 1*: 455–473.

Nader, M. A., Morgan, D., Gage, H. D., Nader, S. H., Calhoun, T. L., Buchheimer, N., et al. (2006). PET imaging of dopamine D2 receptors during chronic cocaine self-administration in monkeys. *Nature Neuroscience, 9* (8): 1050–1056.

Nagel, T. (1974). What is it like to be a bat? *Philosophical Review, 83*: 435–450.

Nardone, I. B., Ward, I., Fotopoulou, A., & Turnbull, O. H. (2007). Attention and emotion in anosognosia: Evidence of implicit awareness and repression? *Neurocase, 13* (5): 438–445.

Nausieda, P., Weiner, W. J., Kaplan, L. R., Weber, S., & Klawans, H. L. (1982). Sleep disruption in the course of chronic levodopa therapy: An early feature of the levodopa psychosis. *Clinical Neuropharmacology, 5*: 183.

Nestler, E. J., & Carlezon, W. A. Jr. (2006). The mesolimbic dopamine reward circuit in depression. *Biological Psychiatry, 59*: 1151–1159.

Nieuwenhuys, R., Voogd, J., & van Huijzen, C. (2008). *The Human Central Nervous System.* New York: Springer.

Nofzinger, E., Mintun, M., Wiseman, M., Kupfer, D., & Moore, R. (1997). Forebrain activation in REM sleep: An FDG PET study. *Brain Research, 770*: 192–201.

Northoff, G. (2011). *Neuropsychoanalysis in Practice: Brain, Self and Objects.* Oxford: Oxford University Press.

Ostow, M. (1954). A psychoanalytic contribution to the study of brain function. 1: The frontal lobes. *Psychoanalytic Quarterly, 23*: 317–338.

Ostow, M. (1955). A psychoanalytic contribution to the study of brain function. 2: The temporal lobes. 3: Synthesis. *Psychoanalytic Quarterly, 24*: 383–423.

Ostow, M. (1962). *Drugs in Psychoanalysis and Psychotherapy.* New York: Basic Books.

Ostow, M. (1980). *The Psychodynamic Approach to Drug Therapy.* New York: Van Nostrand Reinhold.

Ostow, M., & Kline, N. S. (1959). The psychic actions of reserpine and chlorpromazine in psychopharmacology frontiers. In: N. S. Kline (Ed.), *Major Problems and Needs in Psychopharmacology Frontiers.* Boston, MA: Little Brown.

Panksepp, J. (1971). Aggression elicited by electrical stimulation of the hypothalamus in albino rats. *Physiology & Behavior, 6* (4): 31 1–16.

Panksepp, J. (1982). Toward a general psychobiological theory of emotions. *Behavioral and Brain Sciences, 5* (3): 407–467.

Panksepp, J. (1985). Mood changes. In: P. Vinken, C. Bruyn, & H. Klawans (Eds.), *Handbook of Clinical Neurology, Vol. 45.* Amsterdam: Elsevier.

Panksepp, J. (1986). The anatomy of emotions. In: R. Plutchik (Ed.), *Emotion: Theory, Research and Experience, Vol. III. Biological Foundations of Emotions* (pp. 91–124). Orlando, FL: Academic Press.

Panksepp, J. (1998a). *Affective Neuroscience: The Foundations of Human and Animal Emotions.* New York: Oxford University Press.

Panksepp, J. (1998b). The periconscious substrates of consciousness: Affective states and the evolutionary origins of the SELF. *Journal of Consciousness Studies, 5*: 566–582.

Panksepp, J. (1999). Emotions as viewed by psychoanalysis and neuroscience: An exercise in consilience. *Neuropsychoanalysis, 1*: 15–38.

Panksepp, J. (2003a). Can anthropomorphic analyses of "separation cries" in other animals inform us about the emotional nature of social loss in humans? *Psychological Reviews, 110*: 376–388.

Panksepp, J. (2003b). Feeling the pain of social loss. *Science, 302*: 237–239.

Panksepp, J. (2005a). Affective consciousness: Core emotional feelings in animals and humans. *Consciousness and Cognition, 14*: 30–80.

Panksepp, J. (2005b). Feelings of social loss: The evolution of pain and the ache of a broken heart. In: R. Ellis & N. Newton (Eds.), *Consciousness & Emotions, Vol. 1* (pp. 23–55). Amsterdam: John Benjamins.

Panksepp, J. (2006). Emotional endophenotypes in evolutionary psychiatry. *Progress in Neuro-Psychopharmacology, 30*: 774–784.

Panksepp, J. (2007). Criteria for basic emotions: Is DISGUST a primary "emotion"? *Cognition & Emotion, 21*: 1819–1828.

Panksepp, J. (2009). The emotional antecedents to the evolution of music and language. *Musicae Scientiae, 13* (2): 229–259.

Panksepp, J. (2011). Cross-species affective neuroscience decoding of the primal affective experiences of humans and related animals. *PLoS ONE, 6*. doi:10.1371/journal.pone.0021236

Panksepp, J., & Biven, L. (2012). *The Archaeology of Mind*. New York: W. W. Norton.

Panksepp, J., Lensing, P., & Bernatzky, G. (1989). Delta and kappa opiate receptor control of separation distress. *Neuroscience Abstracts, 15*: 845.

Panksepp, J., & Moskal, J. (2008). Dopamine and SEEKING: Subcortical "reward" systems and appetitive urges. In: A. Elliot (Ed.), *Handbook of Approach and Avoidance Motivation* (pp. 67–87). Mahwah, NJ: Lawrence Erlbaum Associates.

Panksepp, J., & Solms, M. (2012). What is neuropsychoanalysis? Clinically relevant studies of the minded brain. *Trends in Cognitive Science, 16*: 6–8.

Panksepp, J. , & Watt, D. F. (2009). Depression: An evolutionarily conserved mechanism to terminate separation distress? A review of aminergic, peptidergic, and neural network perspectives. *Neuropsychoanalysis, 11*: 7–51.

Panksepp, J., Yates, G., Ikemoto, S., & Nelson, E. (1991). Simple ethological models of depression: Social-isolation induced "despair" in chicks and mice. In: B. Olivier & J. Moss (Eds.), *Animal Models in Psychopharmacology* (pp. 161–181). Holland: Duphar.

Pantelis, E., & Solms, M. (2007). *Subjective Correlates of Manipulation of Neuropeptide Systems Relevant to Depression*. Oral presentation to the Hope for Depression Research Foundation Inaugural Symposium, Hotel Imperial, Vienna.

Partridge, M. (1950). *Pre-Frontal Leucotomy: A Survey of 300 Cases Personally Followed for 1½–3 Years*. Oxford: Blackwell.

Parvizi, J., & Damasio, A. R. (2003). Neuroanatomical correlates of brainstem coma. *Brain, 126*: 1524–1536.

Peled, A. (2008). *Bridging the Gap Between Neuroscience, Psychoanalysis and Psychiatry.* Hove: Routledge,

Penfield, W. (1938). The cerebral cortex in man. I: The cerebral cortex and consciousness. *Archives of Neurology & Psychiatry, 40*: 417.

Penfield, W., & Boldrey, E. (1937). Somatic motor and sensory representation in the cerebral cortex of man as studied by electrical stimulation. *Brain, 60*: 389–443.

Penfield, W., & Erickson, T. (1941). *Epilepsy and Cerebral Localization.* Springfield, IL: Charles C Thomas.

Penfield, W., & Jasper, H. (1954). *Epilepsy and the Functional Anatomy of the Human Brain.* Oxford: Little & Brown.

Penfield, W., & Rasmussen, T. (1950). *The Cerebral Cortex of Man: A Clinical Study of Localization of Function.* New York: Macmillan.

Perogamvros, L., & Schwartz, S. (2012). The roles of the reward system in sleep and dreaming. *Neuroscience & Biobehavioral Reviews, 36*: 1934–1951.

Petkova, A., & Ehrsson, H. E. (2008). If I were you: Perceptual illusion of body swapping. *PLoS ONE, 3*. doi:10.1371/journal.pone.0003832

Pfaff, D. W. (1999). *Drive: Neurobiological and Molecular Mechanisms of Sexual Motivation.* Cambridge, MA: MIT Press.

Pfaff, D. W. (2006). *Brain Arousal and Information Theory.* Cambridge, MA: Harvard University Press.

Pompeiano, O. (1979). Cholinergic activation of reticular and vestibular mechanisms controlling posture and eye movements. In: J. A. Hobson & N. Brazier (Eds.), *The Reticular Formation Revisited.* New York: Raven.

Posner, M. I., Cohen, Y., & Rafal, R. D. (1982). Neural systems control of spatial orienting. *Philosophical Transactions of the Royal Society of London Series B. Biological Sciences, 298*: 187–198.

Pryce, C. R., Ruedi-Bettschen, D., Dettling, A. C., Weston, A., Russig, H., Ferger, B., et al. (2005). Long-term effects of early-life environmental manipulations in rodents and primates: Potential animal models in depression research. *Neuroscience and Biobehavioral Reviews, 29*: 649–674.

Ramachandran, V. S., & Blakeslee, S. (1998). *Phantoms in the Brain: Human Nature and the Architecture of the Mind.* London: Fourth Estate.

Ramus, F. (2013). What's the point of neuropsychoanalysis? *British Journal of Psychiatry, 203*: 170–171.

Rizzolatti, G., Fadiga, L., Gallese, V., & Fogassi, L. (1996). Premotor cortex and the recognition of motor actions. *Cognitive Brain Research, 3*: 131–141.

Robinson, T. E., & Berridge, K. C. (2003). Addiction. *Annual Review of Psychology, 54* (1): 25–53.

Rolls, E. T. (1999). *The Brain and Emotion.* Oxford: Oxford University Press.

Sacks, O. (1985). *The Man Who Mistook His Wife for a Hat.* London; Duckworth

Sacks, O. (1990). *Awakenings.* New York: HarperCollins.

Sacks, O. (1991). Neurological dreams. *MD* (February): 29–32.

Sacks, O. (1998). *A Leg To Stand On.* New York: Simon & Shuster.

Sacktor, T. (2008). PKMzeta, LTP maintenance, and the dynamic molecular biology of memory storage. *Progress in Brain Research, 169*: 27–40.

Schacter, D. L. (1996). *Searching for Memory.* New York: Basic Books.

Schacter, D. L., Norman, K. A., & Koutstaal, W. (1998). The cognitive neuroscience of memory. *Annual Review of Psychology, 49*: 289–318.

Scharf, B., Moscovitz, C., Lupton, C., & Klawans, H. (1978). Dream phenomena induced by chronic levodopa therapy. *Journal of Neural Transmission, 43*: 143.

Schilder, P. (2007). *Brain and Personality: Studies in the Psychological Aspects of Cerebral Neuropathology and the Neuropsychiatric Aspects of the Motility of Schizophrenics.* Whitefish, MT: Kessinger.

Schildkraut, J. (1965). The catecholamine hypothesis of affective disorders: A review of supportive evidence. *American Journal of Psychiatry, 122*: 509–522.

Schindler, R. (1953). Das Traumleben der Leukotomierten. *Wiener Zeitschrift für Nervenheilkunde, 6*: 330.

Scoville, W. B., & Milner, B. (1957). Loss of recent memory after bilateral hippocampal lesions. *Journal of Neurology, Neurosurgery and Psychiatry, 20*: 11–21.

Searle, J. R. (1980). Minds, brains and programs. *Behavioral and Brain Sciences, 3*: 417–457.

Shallice, T. (1988). *From Neuropsychology to Mental Structure.* Cambridge: Cambridge University Press.

Shepard, R., & Metzler, J. (1971). Mental rotation of three dimensional objects. *Science, 171*: 701–703.

Shevrin, H., Bond, J. A., Brakel, L. A., Hertel, R. K., & Williams, W. J. (1996). *Conscious and Unconscious Processes: Psychodynamic, Cognitive and Neurophysiological Convergences.* New York: Guilford Press.

Shewmon, D., Holmse, D., & Byrne, P. (1999). Consciousness in congenitally decorticate children: Developmental vegetative state as a self-fulfilling prophecy. *Developmental Medicine & Child Neurology, 41*: 364–374.

Siegel, A. M. (1996). *Heinz Kohut and the Psychology of the Self.* Makers of Modern Psychotherapy Series. London: Routledge.

Solms, M. (1995). New findings on the neurological organization of dreaming: Implications for psychoanalysis. *Psychoanalytic Quarterly, 64*: 43–67.

Solms, M. (1996). Towards an anatomy of the unconscious. *Journal of Clinical Psychoanalysis, 5*: 331–367.

Solms, M. (1997a). What is consciousness? *Journal of the American Psychoanalytic Association, 45*: 681–703.

Solms, M. (1997b). *The Neuropsychology of Dreams: A Clinico-Anatomical Study.* Institute for Research in Behavioral Neuroscience Monograph Series, No. 7. Mawah, NJ: Erlbaum.

Solms, M. (1998a). Before and after Freud's "Project". In: R. Bilder & F.

LeFever (Eds.), *Neuroscience of the Mind on the Centennial of Freud's "Project for a Scientific Psychology"*. *Annals of the New York Academy of Sciences, 843*: 1–10.

Solms, M. (1998b). Psychoanalytische Beobachtungen an vier Patienten mit ventromesialen Frontalhirnlasionen. *Psyche, 52*: 919–962.

Solms, M. (1999). The deep psychological functions of the right cerebral hemisphere. *British Psychoanalytical Society Bulletin, 35* (1): 9–29.

Solms, M. (2000a). Dreaming and REM sleep are controlled by different brain mechanisms. *Behavioral & Brain Sciences, 23*: 843–850.

Solms, M. (2000b). A psychoanalytic contribution to contemporary neuroscience. In: M. Velmans, M. (Ed.), *Investigating Phenomonenal Consciousness: New Methodologies and Maps* (pp. 67–95). Advances in Consciousness Research Series. Philadelphia, PA: John Benjamins.

Solms, M. (2001a). An example of neuro-psychoanalytic research: Korsakoff's syndrome. *Bulletin of the British Psychoanalytical Society, 37* (5): 24–32.

Solms, M. (2001b). *The Interpretation of Dreams* and the neurosciences. *Psychoanalysis and History, 3*: 79–91.

Solms, M. (2002). An introduction to the neuroscientific works of Sigmund Freud. In: G. van de Vijver & F. Geerardyn (Eds.), *The Pre-Psychoanalaytic Writings of Sigmund Freud*. London: Karnac.

Solms, M. (2006). Sigmund Freud Heute: Eine neurowissenschaftliche Perspektive auf die Psychoanalyse. *Psyche, 60*: 829–859.

Solms, M. (2007). *The Interpretation of Dreams* and the neurosciences. In: L. Mayes, P. Fonagy & M. Target (Eds.), *Developmental Science and Psychoanalysis: Integration and Innovation* (pp. 141–158). London: Karnac.

Solms, M. (2011). Neurobiology and the neurological basis of dreaming. In: P. Montagna & S. Chokroverty (Eds.), *Handbook of Clinical Neurology, 98: Sleep Disorders—Part 1* (pp. 519–544). New York: Elsevier.

Solms, M. (2012). Freud, Sigmund. In: D. Barrett & P. McNamara (Eds.), *Encyclopedia of Sleep and Dreams: The Evolution, Function, Nature, and Mysteries of Slumber, Vol. 1* (pp. 290–291). Santa Barbara, CA: Greenwood.

Solms, M. (2013). The conscious id. *Neuropsychoanalysis, 15*: 5–19.

Solms, M. (in press). Reconsolidation: Turning consciousness into memory. *Behavioral & Brain Sciences*.

Solms, M., & Nersessian, E. (1999). Freud's theory of affect: Questions for neuroscience. *Neuropsychoanalysis, 1* (1): 5–14.

Solms, M., & Panksepp, J. (2010). Why depression feels bad. In: E. Perry, D Collerton, F. LeBeau, & H. Ashton (Eds.), *New Horizons in the Neuroscience of Consciousness*. Philadelphia, PA: John Benjamins.

Solms, M., & Panksepp, J. (2012). The id knows more than the ego admits *Brain Sciences, 2*: 147–175.

Solms, M., Pantelis, E., & Panksepp, J. (2012). Neuropsychoanalytic notes on addiction. In: G. Ellis, D. Stein, E. Meintjies, & K. Thomas (Eds.)

Substance Use and Abuse in South Africa (pp. 175–184). Cape Town: University of Cape Town Press.

Solms, M., & Saling, M. (1986). On psychoanalysis and neuroscience: Freud's attitude to the localizationist tradition. *International Journal of Psychoanalysis, 67*: 397–416.

Solms, M., & Turnbull, O. (2002). *The Brain and The Inner World: An Introduction to the Neuroscience of Subjective Experience.* New York: Other Press.

Strawson, G. (1994). *Mental Reality.* Cambridge, MA: MIT Press.

Sulloway, F. J. (1979). *Freud: Biologist of the Mind.* Bungay: Chaucer Press.

Sur, M., & Rubenstein, J. L. R. (2005). Patterning and plasticity of the cerebral cortex. *Science, 310*: 805–810.

Sutton, S., Braren, M., Zubin, J., & John, E. R. (1965). Evoked-potential correlates of stimulus uncertainty. *Science, 150* (3700): 1187–1188.

Sutton, S., Tueting, P., Zubin, J., & John, E. R. (1967). Information delivery and the sensory evoked potential. *Science, 155* (3768): 1436–1439.

Tenore, P. L. (2008). Psychotherapeutic benefits of opioid agonist therapy. *Journal of Addictive Diseases, 27* (3): 49–65.

Tondowski, M., Kovacs, Z., Morin, C., & Turnbull, O. H. (2007). Hemispheric asymmetry and the diversity of emotional experience in anosognosia. *Neuropsychoanalysis, 9*: 67–81.

Tronson, N., & Taylor, J. (2007). Molecular mechanisms of memory reconsolidation. *Nature Reviews. Neuroscience, 8*: 262–275.

Tulving, E. (2002). Episodic memory: From mind to brain. *Annual Review of Psychology, 53*: 1–25.

Turnbull, O. (2001). The neuropsychology that would have interested Freud most. *Neuropsychoanalysis, 3* (1): 33–38.

Turnbull, O. (2004). Founders of neuro-psychoanalysis: Interview with Mortimer Ostow. *Neuropsychoanalysis, 6* (2): 209–216.

Turnbull, O., Berry, H., & Evans, C. E. Y. (2004). A positive emotional bias in confabulatory false beliefs about place. *Brain & Cognition, 55*: 490–494.

Turnbull, O., Evans, C. E. Y., & Owen, V. (2005). Negative emotions and anosognosia. *Cortex, 41*: 67–75.

Turnbull, O., Fotopoulou, K., & Solms, M. (in press). Anosognosia as motivated unawareness: The "defence" hypothesis revisited. *Cortex.*

Turnbull, O., Jenkins, S., & Rowley, M. L. (2004). The pleasantness of false beliefs: An emotion-based account of confabulations. *Neuropsychoanalysis, 6* (1): 5–16.

Turnbull, O., Jones, K., & Reed-Screen, J. (2002). Implicit awareness of deficit in anosognosia: An emotion-based account of denial of deficit. *Neuropsychoanalysis, 4*: 69–86.

Turnbull, O., Owen, V., & Evans, C. E. Y. (2005). Negative emotions in anosognosia. *Cortex, 41*: 67–75.

Turnbull, O., & Solms, M. (2003). Depth psychological consequences of brain damage. In: J. Panksepp (Ed.), *A Textbook of Biological Psychiatry* (pp. 571–596). New York: Wiley.

Turnbull, O., & Solms, M. (2007). Awareness, desire, and false beliefs: Freud in the light of modern neuropsychology. *Cortex, 43*: 1083–1090.

Vandekerckhove, M., & Panksepp, J. (2009). The flow of anoetic to noetic and autonoetic consciousness: A vision of unknowing (anoetic) and knowing (noetic) consciousness in the remembrance of things past and imagined futures. *Consciousness and Cognition, 18*: 1018–1028.

Vogel, G., Barrowclough, B., & Giesler, D. (1972). Limited discriminability of REM and sleep onset reports and its psychiatric implications. *Archives of General Psychiatry, 26*: 449.

Volkow, N. D, Fowler, J. S., Wang, G. J., Hitzemann, R., Logan, J., Schlyer, D. J., et al. (1993). Decreased dopamine D2 receptor availability is associated with reduced frontal metabolism in cocaine abusers. *Synapse, 14* (2): 169–177.

Volkow, N. D., Fowler, J. S., Wang, G. J., & Swanson, J. M. (2004). Dopamine in drug abuse and addiction: Results from imaging studies and treatment implications. *Molecular Psychiatry, 9* (6): 557–569.

Volkow, N. D., Fowler, J. S., Wang, G., Swanson, J. M., & Telang, F. (2007). Dopamine in drug abuse and addiction: Results of imaging studies and treatment implications. *Archives of Neurology, 64* (11): 1575–1579.

Volkow, N. D., Fowler, J. S., Wolf, A. P., Schlyer, D., Shiue, C. Y., Alpert, R., et al. (1990). Effects of chronic cocaine abuse on postsynaptic dopamine receptors. *American Journal of Psychiatry, 147* (6): 719–724.

Volkow, N. D, Wang, G., Begleiter, H., Porjesz, B., Fowler, J. S., Telang, F., et al. (2006). High levels of dopamine D2 receptors in unaffected members of alcoholic families: Possible protective factors. *Archives of General Psychiatry, 63* (9): 999–1008.

Walter, W. G., Cooper, R., Aldridge, V. J., McCallum, W. C., & Winter, A. L. (1964). Contingent negative variation: An electric sign of sensorimotor association and expectancy in the human brain. *Nature, 203*: 320–384.

Watson, J. D., & Crick, F. H. C. (1953). Molecular structure of nucleic acids: A structure for deoxyribose nucleic acid. *Nature, 171*: 737–738.

Watt, D. F., & Pincus, D. I. (2004). Neural substrates of consciousness: Implications for clinical psychiatry. In: J. Panksepp (Ed.), *Textbook of Biological Psychiatry*. Hoboken, NJ: Wiley.

Weinstein, E. A., & Kahn, R. L. (1955). *Denial of Illness: Symbolic and Physiological Aspects*. Springfield, IL: Charles C Thomas.

Winnicott, D. W. (1960). The theory of the parent–infant relationship. *International Journal of Psychoanalysis, 41*: 585–595.

Wright, J., & Panksepp, J. (2012). An evolutionary framework to understand foraging, wanting, and desire: The neuropsychology of the SEEKING System. *Neuropsychoanalysis, 14*: 5–39.

Zeki, S. (1993). *A Vision of the Brain*. Oxford: Blackwell.

Zupancic, M., & Guilleminault, C. (2006). Agomelatine: A preliminary review of a new antidepressant. *CNS Drugs, 20*: 981–992.

INDEX

Printed in the United States
by Baker & Taylor Publisher Services

Printed in the United States
by Baker & Taylor Publisher Services